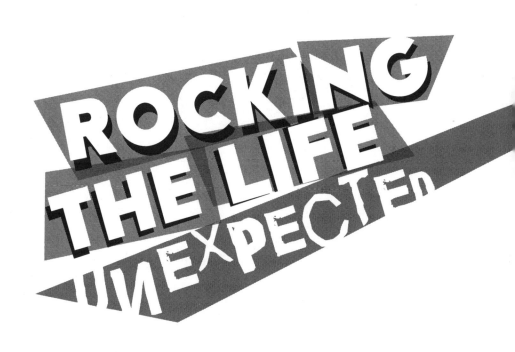

12 Weeks to Your Plan B for a Meaningful
and Fulfiling Life Without Children

Jody Day

Founder of Gateway Women

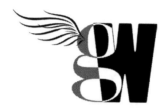

Rocking the Life Unexpected:
12 Weeks to Your Plan B for a Meaningful and Fulfiling Life Without Children

by Jody Day

Founder, Gateway Women www.gateway-women.com

Cover design and Gateway Women logo by Ilona Tofahrn-Flint (ilona@redgrafik.co.uk)

Cover photo: WASP pilots in front of B-17 Flying Fortress bomber.
Lockbourne Army Air Force base, Ohio. (USAF Neg:160449AC, USAF Museum)

Author photograph by Simon Fairclough

Book design by Raj (graphicstudio.raj@gmail.com)

Media Agent: chloe-cunningham@gmail.com

This book includes the author's personal account of dealing with infertility, childlessness and grief, as well as some of the experiences of other women that she has learned about. Any personal information in this book other than the authors has been used with permission. This book is for educational purposes. It is not intended to replace medical advice or the services of a trained professional, physician, support group or other helping professional. This book is sold with the understanding that the publisher and author are not rendering individual psychological or medical services, or individual services of any kind, to the reader. Should such services be necessary, please consult an appropriate professional.

Published by CreateSpace, USA.
ISBN-13: 978-1493607273

This book is dedicated with love to my mother, Elly.

CONTENTS

INTRODUCTION

In this book, we're going to go on a surprising journey together into the past and how you got here, the present you never planned for and a future better than you expected. It's going to be quite a big trip!

> This book is written by a woman who wanted to be a mother and it didn't work out. And that, as you know, is a whole book in itself!

You'll be pleased to know that this book isn't going to tell you to 'get over it', point out that your childlessness isn't actually 'that big a deal', remind you 'how lucky you are that you don't have children', or even suggest that you explore adoption as your obvious next step. Because the fact is, we've all heard variations on these themes far too often. Whilst mothers and others rarely *mean* to hurt our feelings or insult our intelligence, they often manage to do so anyway…

This book is about what I learned as I pulled myself from the pit of despair I felt around my childlessness, and how I found a way to make my life feel meaningful again. It's about the programme I created so that I could share that experience with other women and guide them as they trod *their* own path out of *their* own swamp.

Recently, I was reminded of a particularly low moment in my life a few years ago when I was feeling deeply unhappy and lost. I was considering whether to take a job working with a voluntary organisation in Kabul, but decided against it in the end because I'd have to start my contract in October and I couldn't face the idea of how cold I'd be in the Afghan winter. You see, I wasn't bothered about getting shot or blown up, but I couldn't cope with the idea of getting cold! Looking back on this now, it's clear to me that I felt my life as a childless woman was so worthless that I didn't think that losing it was such a big deal. After all, it's not like my kids and husband needed me, did they? I'd already lost my husband to addiction (no, he didn't die, but he was lost anyway) and I was beginning to realise at the age of 42 that it was increasingly unlikely that I was ever going to become a mother.

Today I love my life again, and being able to guide and support other women as they learn to love *theirs* again brings me great joy and satisfaction. If I had my time over again, I'd still wish to be a mother, but these days I'm genuinely fine with the way things have turned out. Really, I'm not faking it! I find I'm able to enjoy the advantages of *not* being a mother, take pleasure in being around other people's children without dying inside, and really look forward to my future again. I call that having a Plan B and this book is going to help you start moving towards yours.

Together, we're going to start creating your Plan B for a meaningful and fulfilling life without children.

Here's to new beginnings.

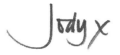

rocking@gateway-women.com

www.gateway-women.com

HOW TO USE THIS BOOK

This book is going to introduce you to some new ways to think and feel about your situation as a childless-by-circumstance woman. It's based very closely on the programme that I've been running since 2011 in London, although I've selected and adapted the exercises to make them a little easier for you to do on your own or as part of your own self-organised reading group. It also contains some entirely new material especially for this book which I've piloted and refined in workshops and working one-to-one with women.

The Gateway Women groups meet weekly for an hour-and-a-half over 12 weeks. Because of the new thoughts and feelings that this work brings up, I recommend that you too might want to read just one chapter each week and then take a break to do the exercises and see what comes up for you. This will give you time to reflect on what you've learned, unlearned and discovered and then integrate that into your new awareness. However, if you prefer to read the book through from beginning to end and do the exercises as you go, or afterwards, I'm sure that will serve you very well too. You might be one of those people who mean to do the exercises but never do (*guilty as charged!*) You'll be missing some of the richness, but do whatever works for you… after all, you're probably fed up of obeying other people's rules anyway!

This book can also be used as a framework to hold your own 12 week reading group with other childless-by-circumstance women in your area. The exercises can be done in the group setting and this can be really powerful – either to see how similar your responses are (when you thought you were the only woman who had those thoughts) or to hear and see new ways of thinking about things that hadn't occurred to you before. Each chapter ends with a 'Reflections' passage, which can act as a helpful conversational starting point for the beginning of each week's group. If you'd like more information on how to host and run a group, check the Gateway Women website.

One thing I really would recommend is that you take the time to fill in the Plan B Healing Inventory which you'll find in the Appendix. You can also print out a copy of this from the Gateway Women website. This will preserve a snapshot of your thoughts and feelings about your situation today and can be a really valuable way to track how this book has changed things for you once you get to the end of the process. However, like everything else in this book, I'd like to stress that this is an *invitation* not an instruction. Part of recovery from childlessness is learning to trust yourself again, so I trust that you'll do what's right for you.

An Overview of this Book s Structure

Although this book has a linear 12 chapter structure, within that structure is an ebb-and-flow between the deeply personal and the more public, societal aspects of being a childless-by-circumstance woman. In working with childless women in groups and workshops, I have found that this structure helps to gently reveal layers of stuck thought and feeling and enables a gradual progression of 'aha' moments that work together in an integrated way.

For some of us, placing our own experience within a broader context helps us to realise that we really aren't the *only* women that 'this has happened to', which can be a huge relief and the start of challenging our shame-based internal monologues. However, for others, this might feel too heady and intellectual and they'd rather dive straight into working with their individual felt experience and come back to some of the societal stuff later.

Because of this structure, you may find that some parts of this book feel more relevant to you right now. So, in order for you to assess this, here is a brief overview of each chapter.

- CHAPTER 1: BEHIND EVERY WOMAN WITHOUT CHILDREN IS A STORY (P. 15)

  The book starts at a very personal level with my story and looks at the power of stories to shape our lives. It explores some of the many different experiences that may have led to us being childless-by-circumstance other than the simplistic 'didn't want' or 'couldn't have' options.

- CHAPTER 2: YOU'RE NOT THE ODD ONE OUT (P. 31)

  We now pull back to survey the broader social and economic context that has led to almost 1:5 women (20%) of our generation reaching 45 without having had children, as opposed to the more historical rate of 1:10 (10%).

- CHAPTER 3: MOTHERHOOD WITH A CAPITAL 'M' (P. 43)

  In this chapter we explore how and why motherhood has become such a minefield of social expectations and pressures for women (both those with and without children). We also begin to examine our own childhood experiences and what messages we may have picked up that have influenced our beliefs and choices around motherhood and childlessness.

- **Chapter 4: Working Through the Grief of Childlessness** (p. 59)

  Grief over childlessness is an issue for us at personal, social and cultural levels, so in this chapter we take a new look at what grief is (and surprisingly, why it's a good thing). We explore how grief impacts us personally, and what we can do to complete our grieving and be ready to embrace our lives again.

- **Chapter 5: Liberating Yourself from the Opinion of Others** (p. 83)

  This chapter pulls back to take a look at the cultural landscape of how, as childless women, we are pigeonholed into a few very reductive and mostly rather unkind stereotypes. We explore why that might be, and what we can do to reframe our experience and choose our *own* labels and celebrate our own role models.

- **Chapter 6: Who Moved my Mojo?** (p. 111)

  For childless-by-circumstance women, the loss of the potential identity of 'mother' can be devastating to our ego and sense of who we are – and thus demolish our mojo, our 'joie de vivre'. This chapter gives insight into why this might be, and how putting 'meaning' back at the centre of our new lives is an important step in getting our mojo back.

- **Chapter 7: Letting Go of Your Burnt Out Dreams** (p. 133)

  Letting go of the dream of motherhood is, for most of us, a very painful experience. In this chapter, we explore what happens when either so much of our life-force was channelled into this dream that other areas of our lives were subjugated, or not enough action was taken due to our struggle with unexamined ambivalence. Either way, our unfulfilled dreams need to be acknowledged, understood, grieved and let go of in order for new dreams to arise.

This chapter looks at how our relationship with our body has been affected by our childlessness, and how for many of us this may have led to a cycle of punishing or disconnecting from our bodies as a way to avoid pain. We explore how healing our relationship to our body can be a powerful route into healing our relationship with life, and ultimately with joy.

We now begin to unpack the relationship we have with ourselves in our head and hearts, and look at the source of some of our shaming and hyper-critical internal dialogues. We learn how becoming a 'good enough mother' to ourselves can be a compassionate and effective way to transform our inner world.

The idea of being 'creative' seems to strike fear into the hearts of many of us, often because we have a very narrow idea of what 'creativity' means. However, without an element of play in our lives, we can feel dead inside. Creativity, play and change. I can feel your fear already… (Please don't skip this chapter!)

Plan B isn't a new job, a new city or a new mantra. It's a fundamental refurbishment of your life from the inside out. In this chapter we debunk some of the myths about your Plan B and introduce you to the forensic tools you'll use to start exploring what your Plan B needs to include to create a life that rocks for *you*. (We also bust the bullshit about why *you personally* can't have a life that rocks!)

- CHAPTER 12: TAKING OFF THE INVISIBILITY CLOAK (P. 235)

It's time to celebrate, collaborate and agitate! In this final chapter we look at ways in which we can come together as childless-by-circumstance women and end our isolation by reaching out and staying connected to each other. We also consider what our wider social influence might be as powerful, connected, liberated, aware, intelligent, independent older women. We consider what our legacy might be if it's not the children we expected to have, and also take a good hard look at our fears about ageing without children.

- APPENDIX (P. 255)

Plan B Healing Inventory – complete this before and after working through this book, or whenever you wish. You will also find a downloadable copy of this on the Gateway Women website at www.gateway-women.com

Online Resources – blogs, websites, forums and other resources from around the world for childless-by-circumstance women. Included in the online resource list at bit.ly/1ca5jEN

Recommended Reading – books that I've read and which have supported me, and others, as we heal from our childlessness and move towards our Plan B. Included in the online resource list at bit.ly/1ca5jEN

Endnotes – references from the text of this book. Included in the online resource list at bit.ly/1ca5jEN

Acknowledgements – a thank you to all of you who have helped make this book possible.

A NOTE ON TERMINOLOGY

In this book, I define 'childless-by-circumstance' (or 'childless') as being without a biological child of your own when you had hoped you would have one someday. It's a harsh phrase, but I don't need to tell *you* how harsh it feels on some days.

I really like the word 'childfree', but this term (or its abbreviation 'CF' or 'CBC' – childfree-by-choice) refers to those women (and men) who have actively *chosen* not to have children. Many of them have insisted since childhood that they didn't want children and have never changed their mind, even though they are often told that they will, 'one day'.

'Childless-by-circumstance' rather than 'childless-by-choice' seems to be the term that describes our situation unambiguously, even though I'm aware that those 'circumstances' can often be fraught with ambiguity!

There are many other terms in use, including the acronym NoMo (not-mother) that I created, and which I'll explore in more depth later in the book. But for now, as you read on, in its simplest terms:

Childless = circumstantial

Childfree = chosen

NoMo = not-mother

ABOUT ME: JODY DAY

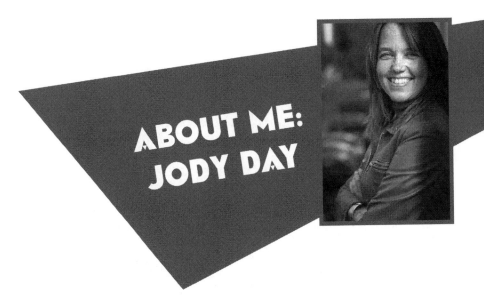

I set up the Gateway Women friendship and support network in London in 2011 with the aim of supporting, inspiring and empowering childless-by-circumstance women like myself to develop meaningful and fulfilling lives without children. It's grown really quickly and I now run groups, workshops, social events and retreats both on and offline as well as giving regular public talks. The private Gateway Women Online Community on G+ started in December 2012 and is growing very quickly with members from all over the English-speaking world. It has already been reviewed as the best online community for childless women. Finally we have our own 'school gates' network!

My own experience of coming to terms with my childlessness was hard, lonely and scary and I wanted to make it easier for other women to make this transition. And I wanted some company too in this new and unexpected part of my life as a childless woman because the loneliness and isolation of being a NoMo (not-mother) in a culture that seems to have gone motherhood-crazy took me completely by surprise.

As Gateway Women has grown and become more influential, I'm increasingly asked to speak in public and am often interviewed in the press. Sometimes I feel like the 'taboo girl' as I've become so comfortable talking about the things that our society still regards as shameful such as medical infertility, social infertility (not having a suitable partner to have children with), menopause, grief and ageing without children. My Plan B turns out to be becoming 'the voice of childless-by-circumstance women' and I love it! Increasingly I'm talking with health-care providers, academics and social policy makers as I'm determined to get our needs and our presence acknowledged, understood and onto the public agenda. As well as what we need, there's also what we have to offer which is often overlooked, not least of all by ourselves.

There's a lot to do to educate people about the stigmas and prejudices we face at present from our friends, families, colleagues, employers, medical professionals, governments and the media. We are 1:5 women turning 45 and with perhaps an even greater number coming up behind us; the time has come for our voice to be heard and our influence to be felt.

It's my mission to get the message out there that it's not only possible to *survive* involuntary childlessness, but to *thrive* as a childless woman and to create a meaningful and fulfilling life without children. I really hope that this book and the support of other Gateway Women helps you to let go of some of your sadness and move towards a life that feels like it fits again. A Plan B that rocks!

Together, we can do this, and more. But first, you have to heal. And for that, you need your sisters. You've found them.

Welcome to your Tribe. Welcome to Gateway Women.

We may not be Mothers,
but we're here,
we care,
we count and
We ROCK

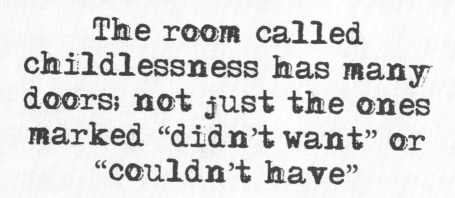

The room called
childlessness has many
doors; not just the ones
marked "didn't want" or
"couldn't have"

CHAPTER I

BEHIND EVERY WOMAN WITHOUT CHILDREN IS A STORY

THIS BOOK IS FOR ALL THE MOTHERS WHO DON'T HAVE CHILDREN.

If you hoped, planned and expected to become a mother one day, but it didn't work out for you, this book is for you.

Wow! What a universe of pain, heartbreak, surprise, dashed hopes, shock and grief are contained in that one short sentence. Pain that the rest of society, our family, colleagues, close friends and often even our partners rarely understand or accept. Or if they do, their concern may come in the form of well-meaning but painful comments or advice that often end up making us feel worse. So we learn that perhaps keeping quiet about our feelings is the safest option.

> 1:5 women in the UK and USA are now reaching their mid-forties without having had children: some of them by choice, many of them by circumstance.

According to the UK Office for National Statistics, 1:5 women born in the UK in the mid 1960s remain childless, compared to 1:9 women born in 1938. That's almost *double* what it was a generation ago.[1] It may be that for the generation born in the 1970s, this will grow further to 1:4 women[2] because of the combined impact of 'social infertility' (being unable to find a suitable partner) coupled with delaying or declining to have children for financial reasons due to the global economic downturn since 2008.

FIFTY WAYS NOT TO BE A MOTHER (WITH APOLOGIES TO PAUL SIMON)

Although most people who don't know our story may imagine that we either chose not to have children or couldn't have them, there are many ways to end up childless without actively choosing it:

1. Being single and unable to find a suitable relationship from your mid-thirties onwards.

2. Being ignorant about your fertility and not realising that after 35 it's half what it was at 25, and that by the time we're 40 we have only a very small number of viable eggs left. The age that many women think they need to worry about is 40, when in fact it's much younger.

3. Not meeting a partner until we're past our childbearing years.

4. Never meeting a suitable partner.

5. Thinking that we don't want children because of our own difficult childhoods, before realising too late that we were not condemned to repeat this with our own children.

6. Being unable to afford to have a child on our own, and being unwilling to rely on the state and therefore risk bringing a child into a life of poverty.

7. Spending our 30s healing childhood wounds in therapy, and then finding it too late to find a healthy partner and start a family.

8. Coming into recovery from addiction issues right at the end of our fertile years.

9. Being with a partner who says they want children later... but the time is never right for them.

10. Being in an emotionally abusive relationship that destroyed our confidence and so we left it too long to leave, recover and find a suitable partner with whom to have children.

11. Not making motherhood a priority and somehow expecting it to 'just happen' one day.

12. Waiting for our partner to come round to the idea of having a family, only to find out that they've decided they definitely don't want children.

13. Infertility issues of our own.

14. Infertility issues of our partner.

15. Infertility issues of both partners.

16. Miscarriage and early term loss.

17. Still birth, cot death, early infancy mortality.

18. Being with a partner who has had a vasectomy and for whom the reversal doesn't work.

19. Coming out of a convent or other seclusion because we want the opportunity to have children, only to be unable to find a partner or to afford to do it on our own.

20. Finding out that the person you'd been in a relationship with for the last few years is actually already married with children.

21. Adopting a child and then finding that although everyone now thinks you're 'a mother', you still feel 'childless' and guilty about it.

22. Staying in a relationship that you don't feel comfortable bringing children into.

23. Trying to conceive for several years only to find out that due to a surgical error a contraceptive coil that should have been removed is still in place.

24. Being widowed.

25. Being born without a fully developed reproductive system.

26. Our own or our partner's sexual orientation leading to relationship breakdown.

27. Not feeling comfortable having IVF or other treatments.

28. Being unable to afford fertility treatments.

29. Not being able to afford to continue fertility treatments.

30. Being denied fertility treatments.

31. Our partner or ourselves being ill during our most fertile years and so waiting for one or both to regain health.

32. Caring for a sick, elderly, disabled or vulnerable family member during our fertile years.

33. Being a 'mother' to our younger siblings in our mother's place (due to illness, absence, death, addiction, depression, etc.) and so believing that we'd 'had enough of mothering' only to realise too late that we would like to have children of our own.

34. Losing a key relationship because of family disapproval on religious, cultural, class, financial or other grounds, and then not meeting another partner in time to start a family.

35. Medical conditions that make becoming a parent difficult.

36. Working in a single-sex dominated environment thus making it difficult to meet a suitable partner.

37. Having genetic inheritance issues of our own, or our partner's, that make us decide not to risk having children.

38. Needing to save enough money to buy a home and pay off college debts before we could afford to start a family, only for it to be too late.

39. Being with a partner who already has children and doesn't want more.

40. Being with a partner who doesn't want children at all (a childfree partner).

41. Becoming a stepmother and for it to be too painful for your partner's children to cope with you having a child.

42. Being unable to get pregnant with the eggs you froze when you were younger.

43. Being ambivalent about motherhood and realising too late that you really do want a family.

44. Finding out that the man who said he wanted children was lying as he'd had a vasectomy and hadn't told you.

45. Having a partner with addiction or mental health issues that took up both of your lives until it was too late to have children.

46. Being unable to adopt because of being single, having insufficient funds, being the wrong age, being the wrong gender, being the wrong ethnicity, being disabled, not being able to afford to or being rejected for a variety of bewildering box-checking reasons including not having a garden!

47. Finding donor egg treatments something you don't feel comfortable pursuing, thereby bringing your fertility treatments to an end.

48. Finding surrogacy as an alternative to having your own baby something you don't feel comfortable with, or can't afford.

49. Having your ovaries damaged by chemotherapy and your partner being unwilling to consider egg donation.

50. Having your surrogate mother decide to keep your genetic child.

I could keep going, but I think you get my point – behind every woman without children is a story, a different one for each of us. Your story may be here, or it may be number 51. I'm sure the list could go on for much longer…

> Most people think that we either chose not to have children or we couldn't. But those of us who are childless-by-circumstance know that that's not the whole story.

My Story

I got married young (although I thought I was very grown-up at the time) at 26. My husband, seven years older than me, was a charming, glamorous fashion designer and we fell madly in love. I wasn't completely sure I wanted children when we married and I told my husband-to-be so; having had a pretty disrupted childhood myself, 'family life' wasn't my idea of fun.

But gradually I got used to the idea, and because it was no longer an abstract idea of 'children', but a child who would be the product of our love and made up of our combined DNA, at 29, we started trying for a family. I had my own PR consultancy by then, but I gave it up to put my skills into helping my husband's new interior design business grow. After all, my thinking went, *his* was the business that was going to support us 'as a family'. Looking back on it now, I can't quite believe how little thought I gave to these decisions; it's like I was following a script and yet if you'd asked me at the time, I would have said that I was an independent thinker.

The interior design business thrived and we worked very well together, but I didn't get pregnant. I wasn't too concerned; I'd had an abortion at 20, which, although it was pretty traumatic emotionally (I was terrified of having a baby as one of the messages I'd internalised from family, school and wider society was that 'children ruin your life') at least it reassured me that everything 'worked'. I was more confused than anything else at my inability to get pregnant because it didn't fit in with my plans – and I was a ferocious planner in those days! I cringe to admit it now but I had a chart listing month-by-month my plans for the next five years of my life, including which months I planned to conceive in so that our children's births would fit around our schedule. I still have that month-by-month planner in a box somewhere; I keep it to remind me how much I've changed, and how I no longer expect life to go according to my plans.

At the age of 33, and four years into trying for a baby, I had a laparoscopy under general anaesthetic – a procedure in which a camera is inserted through your navel to take a look around the reproductive system. 'Ready to move into!' said my avuncular gynaecologist as I came round from the anaesthetic, 'Excellent property! Nothing to worry about!' All the tests on hormones, sperm counts, etc. came back fine too. Looking back on it now, I can't quite believe that after trying to conceive for four years, IVF wasn't even mentioned to us by the doctors, nor was I given any advice about the fact that I only had two years left before I turned 35 and my fertility statistically fell off a cliff. They reassured us that everything was fine, that there was no damage from the abortion, and I was happy to take that at face value.

Over the coming years, we kept on trying (the only advice we ever got from doctors) and meanwhile I saw every nutritionist, herbalist, acupuncturist, shaman, healer, homoeopath, naturopath and quack in London. I tried every diet, made all the lifestyle changes and became an expert on my ovulation dates, peeing on every colour and type of stick you could buy. Yet, each month, regular as clockwork, my period would come and I'd be in tears, yet again.

The doctors called it 'unexplained infertility' and left it at that, never mentioning that we may have been eligible for one or two rounds of IVF treatment paid for by our local health authority. We briefly considered IVF, but couldn't afford it privately and I was very wary of it too – I really didn't like the idea of the hormone treatments and I was convinced I'd conceive naturally anyway. I mean *absolutely, unshakably convinced.* All these years later and with the benefit of hindsight, I can see that my earlier ambivalence over having a family may have found a new home – in my anti-IVF stance. And by the time I *was* ready to consider IVF, at 37, our marriage was not just on the rocks; it was most of the way up the beach. My husband's dashing personality had tipped over into chronic alcoholism and addiction and our lives had become hell. At 38, our marriage was over.

Astonishingly, I still thought there was plenty of time left for me to have a family! I reasoned that because I was young-looking for my age, that my periods were regular as clockwork and that I felt myself ovulating every month, *it must have been my husband.*

On a conscious level, I gave it no more thought and set my mind to getting divorced as quickly as possible and moving on. However, looking back, I can see that perhaps the subconscious pressure of babymania was pushing me to take fast, drastic action. I wonder now, had I not been so desperate for a child, if I would have stayed with my husband and fought for the marriage. But then again, fighting against addiction is never a fairly matched game, and I doubt I would have won. But as all childless-by-circumstance women know, we always wonder how things would have turned out if…

Around the age of 40, I started dating again, and just before my 41st birthday, my ex-husband got a casual girlfriend accidentally pregnant. She either didn't keep the baby or had a very early miscarriage – I can't remember now, the details are hazy with distress. But I do recall how the knowledge of this absolutely devastated me because I could no longer hold onto the fantasy that somehow things were going to work out 'naturally' for me.

In the next few years I had a couple of serious relationships, but sadly neither of them were stable enough to consider doing IVF. And so, when my most serious post-divorce relationship ended, I was 43 years old. Well, 43½ actually!

I remember a gloomy, rainy February afternoon in the tiny, grotty studio-flat I'd rented. I'd moved there a couple of weeks earlier after a stormy and distressing breakup. I was standing watching the rain on the window when the traffic in the street seemed to become completely muted. In that moment, I became acutely aware of myself, standing there, looking out of the window. And then it came to me:

It's over. I'm never going to have a baby.

I realised with absolute clarity and complete certainty that even if I *were* to meet a new partner immediately, we'd need to be together for at least a year before we could even *think* about doing IVF. It was too late for that. I was too old.

It was over. I was never going to have a baby.

But instead of falling apart, something remarkable happened. *I fell together.*

These days, I feel comfortable calling it an epiphany. It started as a strong physical sensation that all the energy I'd been using to run the two separate 'versions' of my life all these years somehow merged back together. It was an odd feeling, as if the 'Jody who had been going to be a mother one day', and who'd been my constant shadow for the last 15 years, reintegrated with the rest of me – the life I was actually living.

Then, another new thought popped up: I thought back to when I'd been 20, and how I used to survey the vast landscape of time ahead of me until I turned 50 and how I imagined that this gave me enough space to achieve whatever I set my sights on. The second new thought said: *If the years from 20 to 50 can feel like that, why can't the years from 45 to 75 feel the same? As long as my health holds out, surely I can achieve something pretty significant in that time?*

I stood still, shocked: *When was the last time I had thought something like that?!*

Over the rest of the day, feelings and thoughts that I hadn't had for years started to bubble up. Amongst the wreckage of my life, I saw the beginnings of a new kind of hope. It was startling because I hadn't been able to imagine a future other than motherhood for such a long time that I'd forgotten it existed. It had been a baby or, well, nothing. A cliff of nothingness that I imagined falling off and hurtling downwards, forever. The few times I *had* imagined alternative futures I'd learned to quash them, fearful that somehow even *thinking* about them would nix my chances of becoming a mother.

I'd love to say that *Halleluiah* I was fixed from that moment forwards. But the truth is that what happened that day is that I came out of denial about my situation. I no longer saw my childlessness as a temporary situation on the way to motherhood, but as a permanent one. I was a childless woman, and would always be so. I am so grateful that I received a hint that day of what lay in my future, as I then entered a period of profound grief for the children I would never have, the life I would never live. But I had no idea it was grief – it would have been a huge help if I'd known.

Soon after I was accepted onto a course to train as a psychotherapist and was due to start my training the following year. It was something I'd wanted to do for almost ten years but had kept putting aside. *Commit to a five-year training? What if I had a baby?* The training, which is ongoing, gave me an opportunity to start processing my sadness, gave me new ways to think about things and new friends to talk about them with.

About a year later, I started writing about being childless in a motherhood-mad world on a new blog I started: Gateway Women. I told it like it was and as I wrote about my situation and had the kind of frank, online discussions with women that I'd been longing to have for years, women from all over the world wrote back and said: *Thank God I'm not the only one… Thank you for finally telling the truth…*

After a lot of encouragement, I gave my first public talk to a tiny audience of eight women, most of whom I knew, and was almost sick with anxiety. A journalist came to the talk and later interviewed me for a national newspaper and before long I was on the radio and in the media regularly. After each bit of publicity, I'd receive loads of emails from women asking for my help. So, with my heart in my mouth and hugely nervous, I started the first Gateway Women group to see if I really could help other women through what I'd been through. Running that group was life-changing for me and for the first few women who attended. I've run it many times now, and I've learned as much as I've taught, thanks to the gutsy, pioneering women who've dared to break the taboo of talking about being childless-by-circumstance. I also run weekend workshops, retreats and give regular public talks and am often in the media as I'm still one of the very few women who is prepared to be named and photographed and to talk openly about being childless.

Not having a family broke my heart. Some may think that's melodramatic, but I know it's true. However, grieving that loss and the life I longed for healed my heart bigger than it was before. It changed me profoundly, and in ways I am still discovering. Five years on from that February afternoon I can say that although the sadness of not being a mother will always be a part of who I am, it no longer defines me.

> I have a future again because the love I had for my unborn children created the grief that healed me.

You never 'get over' childlessness – but it is possible to heal around it. My childlessness was once an open wound and getting through the days was as much as I could do; I was the walking wounded. Now that wound has healed into a scar and I can live with a scar, dance with a scar, dream with a scar. It's a part of me now, though it will always be a tender spot. I loved my unborn children and they will always be with me, but now my life goes forward with them safely inside my heart forever.

My unborn children gave me the gift of love, even though we never met.

WHY OUR STORIES MATTER

Throughout human history, stories have been the way that information has been remembered, honoured and passed on. Before we were able to record stories in writing, storytelling was the only way that a community's history and culture could be handed down.

> Who we are, and who we believe ourselves to be is, to a huge degree, the result of the stories we tell ourselves.

We may think that our memory is accurate, but it is highly selective, like the editor of a news channel. If the data doesn't fit 'our story' we may choose not to notice it or, if we do notice it, to discount, diminish or forget it. Indeed, recent experiments in neuroscience have shown that 'the more often you remember something, the less accurate the memory becomes.'[3]

As childless women, our stories are currently invisible – our individual experience seems to exist in a cultural vacuum. In vain, we look for our reflection in films, books, on TV and in magazines, but we're not there. Or if we are, it's probably as a sad first-person confessional, a social commentary about the impending demographic disaster of an ageing population, or as a warning to younger women to get pregnant as soon as possible (if only it were that simple!) Women around the age of 40 still hoping to have a family are routinely either pitied or ridiculed whilst older childless women are disregarded or mistrusted. The true complexity of our lives as childless women and the many different doors we came through to arrive in this room together are glossed over. As are the positive and hopeful stories of women (and couples) who have not just survived this difficult experience but moved forward in ways that feel meaningful to them.

It is absolutely vital for our sanity and sense of belonging that our stories be heard – the taboo that has kept us silent in the past needs to be dismantled one story at a time, one woman at a time. 1:5 women turning 45 doesn't have children, so we are hardly a minority anymore. However, whereas childfree women are beginning to be heard (they tend not to feel so self-conscious or ashamed about their situation as it was a choice they made freely), childless-by-circumstance women are still misunderstood and misrepresented. As the poet Muriel Rukeyser wrote: *The universe is made of stories, not of atoms.*[4]

All memories are stories (and not the incontrovertible 'facts' we often convince ourselves) and they shift over time, just as stories do.

> The power of stories is that they can recreate old worlds or create new ones. They have the power to transform our reality, even our memories and with that, our beliefs.

I have learned that through telling our stories to each other as childless women and then by examining some of the ways we've chosen to interpret our story (often by using some of the dominant narratives of our time – success/failure, smart/dumb choices, etc.) we can begin to shift our perception. With support and recognition, we can let go of the feeling of being victimised by our circumstances and begin to see the benefits and opportunities they bring. (*Yeah, right,* I heard you say!) In doing so, we can create a story that makes more sense to us right now, one which supports us as we create a fulfilling and meaningful future; one that serves us and other childless women.

Stories touch us, move us, change us. Telling our stories, hearing others' stories and finally feeling heard, changes us too.

EXERCISE 1: YOUR STORY

What is your story about how you came to be a woman without children?

Write it out twice. About 800-1000 words is suggested, but do what feels right for you. Write it once in the 'first person' and once again in the 'third person'.

Once you've written both versions, take some time to reflect on it – some of the following points may help:

- Notice if you share different details in writing your story from these two different perspectives.

- Is there one version of your story that you feel more comfortable with and, if so, what do you think that's about?

- Does either of these stories sound like the story you tell when someone genuinely wants to know the background to your situation? Or is the story you share a more sanitised or over-dramatised version?

- Did you remember parts of your story that you hadn't thought about in a while… or did you realise that you've changed the details over time?

- How do you feel now you've written it all down?

- Keep your stories in a safe place – you may find it interesting to read them in a few years' time to see how things have shifted for you.

REFLECTIONS ON THIS CHAPTER

Take a moment to reflect on how the last week has been for you, or however long it's been since you worked through Chapter 1. Have you noticed any new thoughts and feelings coming up?

What was it like for you to write down your story? Was it good to get it down on paper and out of your head, or did you struggle with it? What did you do with your story once you'd written it? Did you share it with others, put it away somewhere for safekeeping or did you destroy it in case someone found it?

There is no right or wrong way to do this exercise. I would just ask you to take a moment to reflect on how it was for you, and to notice and honour whatever comes up.

By sharing my story, many other women have recognised elements of their own story within it, and have thus been encouraged to share theirs. And then others have found elements in their story, which in turn has inspired them to open up. This is how change begins—by telling our stories.

We are all carrying so much shame attached to our stories, but when we hear others tell theirs and begin to notice that we don't automatically think badly of them for how things turned out, we begin to consider easing up on ourselves. And once the energy formerly used in beating ourselves up starts going towards healing and growing… well, it creates a space for new things to start happening. It doesn't matter how small the shift is, it's the start that matters. It's like the 'trim tab', that small flap on the rudder of an ocean liner or an aeroplane wing which moves first, and in doing so creates a tiny change in flow that makes possible a big change in direction.

Small changes can have a very big effect!

Life is **long** but
fertility is short.

CHAPTER 2

YOU'RE NOT THE ODD ONE OUT

YOU'RE NOT THE ODD ONE OUT

Although when you look around you in the street, amongst your friends and family or in the media you may sometimes feel like the *only* woman who isn't a mother, the surprising fact is that 1:5 women are currently reaching their mid-forties without having had children.[5] *So where the hell are they all then?* We'll get to that later!

The last time the rate of childlessness was this high in the population was for women born around 1900. Research has shown that this was due to two factors: the large number of women who remained unmarried due to the loss of so many men in the First World War, and the effect of the Great Depression of the 1930s on both fertility and finances.[6] Rather shockingly these were known as the 'surplus women'.[7]

The fact that it took the most devastating war this world has seen in terms of loss of life, coupled with the Great Depression, to suppress birth rates to this same extent before shows that we are indeed living through a period of massive social change. It really isn't 'just us'.

Your Story in Context:
The Shock Absorber Generation

I call the generation of women (and men) who were born in the 1960s and 1970s to mothers who hadn't had the same easy access to birth control, higher education and professional careers that we did the 'shock absorber generation for the sexual revolution'.

When I was growing up my mother, who'd had me at 18 'out of wedlock' (as it was called in those days) married unhappily whilst I was still a toddler in order to provide a 'respectable' home for me. Growing up, she instilled in me the belief that a life *outside* the domestic sphere was the one to aspire to, and that education and ambition were important. As far as I can recall, she never once suggested to me that when I grew up I should get married and have a family.

Now, I'm not saying that *every* 60s and 70s mother would have given the same message – but I've spoken to enough childless women aged 40 and over to know that many of us can identify with this. However, like all aspects of circumstantial childlessness, a great deal more research needs to be done.

Although the contraceptive pill was made available on the NHS (the British health service) in 1961[8], my Catholic-raised mother knew so little about how babies were made that she didn't even know she needed to use contraception, and hence my unscheduled arrival in 1964.

Whilst my mother never told me *not* to have children, she made it pretty clear that there were other options that were *more* interesting, meaningful and liberating for me to aspire to. When I became sexually active as a teenager, she encouraged me to go on the pill immediately. She also taught me the facts of life so early (I think I was about eight) that I really didn't have a clue what she was talking about! Her love for me included protecting me from what had happened to her.

Many men who've grown up with similarly frustrated mothers also picked up that having a family 'traps' you. This, reinforced by the fact that women don't need the kind of financial support they used to, contributes to many of them feeling that they don't have to make the kind of early and long-term commitments they used to. If women can have children out of marriage and it's no longer a 'sin'; if you don't 'have' to marry a woman if you 'get her pregnant' and if sex doesn't automatically run the risk of pregnancy, where's the urgency for men to 'settle down' these days? They can remain 'free' for as long as they want and many are choosing to do so. There's also not the same status to being a 'family man' that there once was – these days it seems that a high disposable income and a good-looking partner seems to have more kudos than the more private sacrifices and satisfactions of family and domestic life.

Perhaps also some men may be reluctant to take on the role of fatherhood having seen so little of their *own* fathers whilst growing up. Combined with his frustrated mother's possible resentment towards her own subservient role and the unspoken (or spoken) resentment she had towards his father, it's not hard to imagine that he might wish to construct his life on an entirely different template.

The old 'marriage deal' isn't really possible any more and its prevalence in the past may actually have been overstated in our current cultural nostalgia for more 'settled' times. Those sole-breadwinner families living in comfortably-sized sized homes maintained by a secure (and well-pensioned) income – they hardly exist anymore. And, as for an uncomplaining and obedient wife, home-cooked meals on the table every night, freedom from domestic chores, children in bed by 7pm, good free state-schooling and a community of non-working women around to share the childcare… it's another world, another age and these days, a lifestyle only available to the very rich. Meanwhile, professionals such as teachers, solicitors and doctors, many of whom in the past were able to afford to live like this on one income, now scrabble to achieve something like it on two incomes, not enough sleep and a mountain of debt.

> The old model is broken, but it shimmers like a mirage in the distance. It's going to take time for us all to accept that it's gone.

The next generation, growing up in such stressed-out families and watching their parents tear themselves apart trying to make it work, will probably choose a very different model to organise *their* own family lives. But the shock absorber generation? We're the ones metabolising the shock of integrating these changes into our culture, and many of us are reeling from the disparity between our lives and the ones we *expected* to be living. And sadly many of us think that's our own fault – and that's certainly the message that mainstream culture reflects back at us.

Since humans evolved, if a man and a woman had sex, it was highly likely that it would lead to a baby. It's important to realise what a complete and absolute game-changer the pill has been in all our lives.

The sexual revolution has enabled women to achieve increased equality in many areas, but not in that of fertility. Life is long, but fertility is short, and as so many of us in the shock absorber generation tried to pack education, career, marriage and babies into our 20s and 30s (with a last dash to the altar of the fertility gods in our early 40s), the disparity between men's and women's fertility has come into stark contrast.

Women have joined a professional working world which has grown up around the male template of working incredibly hard to establish your career in your 20s and 30s and to delay starting a family until your 40s – a model which runs counter to female fertility. Sadly, this is something that many of us who are childless-by-circumstance have found out the hard way.

In 2012, University of Huddersfield psychologist Kirsty Budds analysed the media rhetoric around 'delayed motherhood' and concluded that:

> *For a lot of women it isn't a selfish choice but is based around careful decisions, careful negotiations and life circumstances such as the right partner and the right financial position. These women are effectively responsibly trying to produce the best situation in which to have children, which is encouraged societally, but then they are chastised because they are giving birth when older, when it is more risky.*[9]

The pill, women's education, and women's wholesale entry into higher education and the professional working world has completely changed the way men and women relate to each other socially, culturally, sexually and as potential parents.

In one generation, we've turned on their head aeons of courtship and mating behaviours, and the 'shock absorber generation' is working this through within the day-to-day lived context of our lives. We're a living experiment.

Hopefully, the generations that come after us will learn from our experiment that 'having it all' is a myth, that lunch isn't 'for wimps' and that equality doesn't necessarily have to mean going head-to-head with men in a working pattern that many of *them* don't like either! Rather, equality should mean that both men *and* women are *equally* entitled to a culture that makes it possible to live balanced, healthy and purposeful lives, whether that involves being a parent or not.

Choice, What Choice?

In 1969 Carol Hanisch's paper 'The Personal is Political'[10] was published and remains a key text today within the feminist movement. And here we are, almost half a century later, fighting for the choice to be mothers.

'Failing' to become a mother, particularly when there are no obvious medical issues, is seen primarily as some kind of 'choice'. Yet for those of us who've lived that choice, we know that it's a damned-if-you-do, damned-if-you-don't kind of choice:

- What choice is it to choose to become a mother with a man you're not sure is going to stick around?

- What choice is it to choose to become a mother when you know that you'll get no help around the home and yet you'll also need to work?

- What choice is it to choose to be a mother when you know that it means either being 'mummy-tracked' or never really getting your career going again?

- What choice is it to choose to become a single mother in a society where childcare can cost almost your whole salary?

- What choice is it to put off motherhood until you (and your partner) can afford to do so, but risk age-related infertility?

Most women I've spoken to feel that their failure to become a mother is because of the poor choices *they've* made and that they should have made different choices:

- That perhaps she should have married 'him' (even though he was a bit nuts).

- That she shouldn't have married 'him' because he was always flaky.

- That she should have come out about her sexuality earlier.

- That she should have spent less time travelling and getting an education and more time hunting for a partner.

- That she should have started internet dating earlier.

- That she should have lost weight, gone blonde, had cosmetic surgery...

- That she should have had the baby she conceived at 20.

- That she should have realised that not everyone is attracted to a highly educated partner.

- That she should have educated herself about her fertility much, much earlier.

- That she shouldn't have listened to her mother, or that she *should* have listened to her mother.

- That she should have moved abroad, or should never have left her home town.

- That she should have been more adventurous, or more cautious.

- That she should have taken better care of herself.

- That she should have frozen her eggs.

- That she should have got pregnant 'accidentally-on-purpose'.

- Etc. The list is endless.

'Should' is an exhausting, finger-wagging word and reaffirms one of the dominant beliefs of our time – that everything in life is down to making the *right choices*. With such a belief driving you, your list of 'should-haves' is one you can rake over indefinitely. And that way lies madness ...

These choices are rock-and-a-hard place choices and fail to take into account the wider socio-cultural environment where we continue to vote for governments that refuse to legislate for family-friendly working environments (actually, people-friendly working environments are what's needed) and a level of practical support that would make parenthood more affordable and egalitarian.

THE SWEDISH EXPERIENCE

The kind of environment that supports women (and men) in their choice to parent is *not* economically impossible, despite what many governments say. They've done it in Sweden and reversed the European-wide post baby-boom drop in birth rates, whilst simultaneously increasing the number of women in the workforce. Sweden has an almost equal number of men and women in the workforce, more women on the boards of top companies than in any other country and an equality in the domestic tasks of childrearing unknown elsewhere in the developed world. The result: a sane, balanced, egalitarian and highly productive economy.[11] They're also a lot less dismissive of the childless and childfree, because parenthood is seen as a part of life, not life itself.

And how did they achieve this feat of social engineering? By making parental allowances (time-off when a baby is born) both generous *and* a requirement that it be shared equally between both parents; by making high-quality, state-provided child-care freely available and providing excellent state education and health care. Yes, they pay for it with a 56.6% rate of income tax, but consider it fair and well spent.[12] However, there are rumblings that perhaps the generation of children brought up this way are not doing so well as young adults, and that Swedish schools are dealing with massively increased levels of bullying, truanting and violence as a result of poorly socialised children.[13] So, as with all social changes, Sweden may now need to deal with the unintended consequences of such changes, and make some adjustments.

So, it can be done. But it may take the huge generational bump of childless-by-circumstance women in the UK, parts of Europe, Australia, Canada and the US to make it happen. Even though it's too late for us, it may yet be our gift to the next generation.

EXERCISE 2: MESSAGES AND CHOICES

Grab a pile of Post-It notes. Write each word or phrase that comes to mind in response to this exercise on a separate Post-It note (or separate small pieces of paper).

Spend a few minutes thinking about some of the 'messages' you picked up when you were a child about dating, mating, marrying and mothering. Some of your messages might include statements such as:

- Men can't be trusted.
- It's a woman's place to compromise.
- Children ruin your life.
- See the world first.
- All men are bastards.
- Motherhood is every woman's destiny.
- Nice girls finish last.
- Men don't want to hear about your feelings.
- Always be financially independent.
- Once you've had a child you're trapped.
- Without a baby you're not complete.
- Unmarried women can't be trusted.
- You made your bed, now lie in it.

- What happens behind closed doors is family business.
- Grab the first partner that comes along.
- If you're not engaged by 30 you're on the shelf.
- Etc., etc…

Once you've written them all out, arrange them on a wall or window and step back to take a look at them as a whole:

- Do they make coherent sense as a whole or do some of them contradict each other?

- Do you still believe these are 'facts' or can you see they might be just opinions, and perhaps not even *your* opinions?

- Reflect on which messages still feel congruent with the person you are today and which ones are past their sell-by date.

- Using this information, reflect on the notion that your 'choices' around relationships and having a family may not have been entirely 'free choices' after all…

REFLECTIONS ON THIS CHAPTER

In this chapter we've taken a galloping tour through the socio-economic and cultural background to the largest increase in childlessness since the First World War and the Great Depression combined. Having taken all that on board, you may find that you are starting to view your story in a new way, both from a personal perspective (your own childhood experience) and also within a broader cultural one.

*Sometimes, placing your own story within the context of the 'shock-absorber generation' theory can change the way you view it. It's also not unusual to feel angry when we realise that our choices (the very ones we've beaten ourselves up about for so very long) were not entirely 'our own' to make, nor the consequences of them quite so much our fault as we, and others, sometimes insist. And yet at other times, knowing that we were not quite the free agents of modernity that we had believed can bring us some relief. It's also possible to feel both angry **and** relieved at the same time!*

*If you did the 'Messages and Choices' exercise, you may have noticed that quite a few of the 'beliefs' you hold (or held) about being a woman, a mother, men, relationships, careers, etc., were often contradictory and that you probably don't even agree with half of them anymore, if you ever fully did. Sometimes it can come as quite a surprise to us when we realise how much credence we've given to messages that, although they may have made **some** sense to us when we were kids (or that we trusted would make sense when we grew up), have remained unexamined and thus active, to this day. Although you may be profoundly upset and regretful to realise that some of your major life decisions have been strongly influenced by beliefs your adult self disagrees with, this is not another reason to give yourself a hard time. But what it **does** mean is that from this point forward, you have the option to choose your beliefs consciously and with great care.*

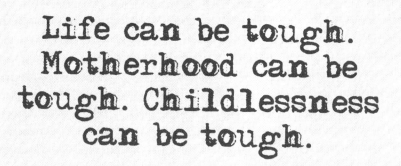

Life can be tough.
Motherhood can be
tough. Childlessness
can be tough.

CHAPTER 3

MOTHERHOOD WITH A CAPITAL 'M'

BEING A MOTHER MEANS

How do you mentally finish that sentence in your mind? Does it include any of the following?

Being a mother means:

- Love
- Nurturing
- Comfort
- Play
- Joy
- Never being alone
- Grandchildren
- Laughter
- Cuddles
- Fulfilment
- Being a real woman
- Etc…

Whilst such things are commonly associated with the joy of motherhood in our culture, for many of us who have been denied that experience, we may erroneously come to believe that many of them are *only* accessible through motherhood.

It isn't true, but it's an overwhelming cultural belief right now. Everywhere you look, motherhood with a capital 'M' is trumpeted as the answer to absolutely everything. This isn't helpful to mothers either as it makes it very hard for them to be open and honest about how tough and unsatisfying it can be to be a mother sometimes.

The good news is that there *are* other ways to access many of the experiences and feelings that you currently associate only with motherhood. Right now, you may be suspicious at this suggestion, but please stay with me! Whilst the experience of being a mother has a uniquely intense quality that we will never know, it is absolutely *not* the only way to access joy, fulfilment, meaning, love, play and many of the other things you might currently feel deprived of.

> Motherhood is not an inoculation against sadness, disappointment, ageing, loss, abandonment, betrayal, disease, old age and death.

The human condition is a struggle for us all – a mixture of joy and sadness, of getting or not getting what we want and losing those things we care about. This is true for all of us, mothers or not.

One of my favourite sayings is from the ancient Greek philosopher Plato who wrote: 'Be kind. For everyone you meet is fighting a hard battle.'[14]

Having children is not a free pass to a happy life. If we look at the lives of mothers without jealousy and listen to them without prejudice, we know this to be true. They suffer too and sometimes their children are the very source of that suffering.

In fact, Rachel Cusk, who wrote a frank memoir of motherhood, 'A Life's Work, On Becoming A Mother'[15] was attacked viciously by the media for daring to tell the truth of her experience and breaking the 'motherhood is meaningful' script. In the reviews of her book there was a level of vitriol that had nothing to do with her book (which was praised by those who could see beyond their outrage) and everything to do with shaming her as a woman and more crucially, as a mother. In a 2008 article for The Guardian she reflects on the pointed, personal and vicious mauling she received upon her book's publication:

> These days I have a better understanding of the intolerance to which, for a while, I fell victim. I see that, like all intolerance, it arose from dependence on an ideal. I see that cruelty and rudeness and viciousness are its harbingers, as they have always been. I see that many – most – of my female detractors continue to write routinely in the press about motherhood and issues relating to children. Their interest in these issues has a fixated quality, compared with their worldly male equivalents.[16]

I remind myself to hold on to mothers who tell the truth like Rachel Cusk when other mothers tell me I'm so 'lucky' I don't have children because I get to travel, sleep in, go out late, do what I want and socialise all the time. In their minds, it's as if we childless women are still irresponsible, carefree twenty-somethings rather than the mature women with serious responsibilities and hefty financial requirements that we are.

For those of us who are single, they also perhaps don't realise that we get no tax-breaks, have no one to split the bills with, and rarely have anything leftover at the end of the month with which to socialise and go on holidays. Indeed, in January 2013 The Atlantic magazine published a detailed analysis by Lisa Arnold and Christina Campbell called 'The High Price of Being Single in America'[17] showing their calculations that over a lifetime, being a single woman as compared to a married one costs between $484,368 to $1,022,096 extra. 'More than a million dollars just for being single', they write. Later in the same article the authors claim that they have 'made only the most conservative of estimates' because they too thought that 'these sums are just too crazy: surely we must have miscalculated or reasoned wrong.'

It seems that even those living the reality of being single (as both the authors of the article are) found their analysis of the data hard to believe beacuse it went against the established belief that single childless women have both money and time to burn and really nothing to moan about. *So will we please shut up?* is the unspoken push-back.

We know that the 'rich and carefree' fantasy that parents have about childless adults isn't true (well, not for most of us anyway), so perhaps we can begin to see that *our* fantasy about the lives of parents may be similarly unreal. Rachel Cusk is one of the very few mothers who has dared to tell the truth of her experience of motherhood to those *not in the know*, yet these are matters which mothers share freely with each other in private. It was not *what* she said, but *who* she said it to that seemed to be the problem. I look forward to the day when we succeed in dismantling the whole 'mummy myth' so that mothers-to-be know what to *really* expect when they're expecting and childless women are not made miserable with the idea that they are only allowed the scraps of life. The fetishisation of motherhood is a fantasy that serves neither groups of women and oppresses both. It also divides women in such a way as to serve the status quo by keeping us squabbling and suspicious of each other, rather than supporting each other as we move forwards to full equality.

> As childless women, part of our journey back to a full and happy life again is beginning to see the whole picture, not just the glossy media fantasy of motherhood. Life can be tough. Motherhood can be tough. Childlessness can be tough.

However, whereas the trials of motherhood are, on the surface, recognised and understood by others, the trials of childlessness seem to be completely invisible and worthless. For all the kindness and empathy we childless women show others around us; for all the understanding and support we give to the mothers in our lives and communities; for all the talk about children and childrearing we sit through politely, unable to contribute – sometimes it seems that the only ones who have any conception of the compromises, difficulties and losses of our own lives are other childless women. Everyone else seems to think we're either making a fuss about nothing or that we're actually really lucky not to have children but too stupid or pathetic to notice.

Such lack of empathy or compassion is also hard to bear when, on a daily basis, we see the impact of women who, whilst they were physically able to bear a child are not psychologically mature enough or well enough or supported enough to parent. Yet, regardless of whether they can parent effectively or not, they are automatically accorded the exalted status of 'mother'. Whereas we childless women, some of us who work with their distressed and disadvantaged offspring, are considered not to be 'real women' somehow. We're seen as a bit of an embarrassment, frankly. Leftover women. And this sucks and makes our situation even harder to bear.

For the Greeks and the Romans to exile someone was a fate worse than death, for they would be cut off from the support of friends, family and civilisation. Sometimes, being a childless woman can feel like that. Like being an unwanted stranger in your own land, not being quite sure what you did wrong to deserve this shaming, this othering.

The Fetishisation of Motherhood

For those of us who wanted to be mothers, it can seem that the whole world has gone absolutely motherhood-mad. When I was growing up in the 1970s, motherhood seemed to be a pretty 'normal' activity for women and nobody made a big deal about it. There was a famous baby book around by an American paediatrician called Dr Spock[18] but there were no designer buggies, no glamorous children's clothes and no 'celebrity bump watch'. The grown-ups did grown-up things, ate grown-up food and seemed to have access to a grown-up world, whilst we children went to bed at 7pm, did chores to earn our pocket money and were often told to leave the grown-ups alone as they were talking. Pregnant women wore maternity smocks to hide their bump, not figure hugging clothes to show it off.

There was nothing note-worthy or celebratory about being pregnant outside the family circle; if anything the impression I got as a child was that being pregnant was one of those slightly embarrassing things that women's bodies did and which you didn't talk about.

Fast forward to the 21st century, and we find a large swathe of (mostly) middle-class women for whom motherhood has become an unattainable dream due to 'social infertility' (not finding a suitable partner) as well as an unaffordable luxury for many couples. And our cultural response? To fetishise the trappings of motherhood.

From the designer buggies to the cult of the yummy mummy and her terrifyingly affluent American cousin, the 'Momzilla'[19] as the writer Jill Kargmen termed her, many of today's middle-class children appear to be treated like precious and breakable artefacts and motherhood seems to have become a competitive and rarefied sport. This is not helpful for mothers, children, wider society or the future.

Whatever can be going on culturally when even a Z-list celebrity can make the front cover of a magazine simply for getting pregnant? It seems that right now, becoming a mother is the most noteworthy and prestigious thing a woman can do. As someone remarked to me recently, if a woman announces her pregnancy on Facebook you'd think she was the first woman ever to conceive, so long is the thread of congratulations.

Now, motherhood is indeed the most important role to *that woman's children*, and parenting has a crucial role to play in society as the route through which the rules and beliefs of the culture are passed on. But it is not fundamentally newsworthy or miraculous. Except at Christmas – a festival celebrating the ultimate miracle baby story!

The current cultural adulation of motherhood, at a time when 1:5 women are reaching the menopause without having had children, is particularly hard on childless-by-circumstance women. It's a role that we will never be able to play and we are also considered not to have a say in it either. A whole new generation is being reared to inhabit and inherit our world and we are considered to have no part in it or influence over it.

> The glorification of motherhood can be explained as what happens when rampant pronatalism meets rampant consumerism.

If 'pronatalism' is a new term to you (it was to me), it's explained by Laura Carroll in her 2012 book 'The Baby Matrix' as:

> *...the idea that parenthood and raising children should be the central focus of every person's adult life. Pronatalism is a strong social force and includes a collection of beliefs so embedded that they have come to be seen as 'true.'*[20]

As Carroll explores, pronatalism is not a new concept – it's been around whenever it's suited the church, state or powers-that-be that expanding the population would cement its power.

But what *is* hard to stomach is that whilst pronatalism is being preached from every pulpit ('be fruitful and multiply') and from the front page of every magazine, there is little political will to create a society that would make it easier for more women to have those children if they could or wished to. I was staggered when I found out that the US, as perhaps currently the most rampantly pronatalist culture, makes no provision whatsoever for paid maternity leave. None. Zero.

One of the dictionary definitions of fetish is 'an object of unreasonably excessive attention or reverence', and also 'an object that is believed to have magical or spiritual powers'. Combining pronatalism with consumerism along with the rise in involuntary childlessness has turned motherhood, children and the trappings of both into a fetish. And this makes being a childless-by-circumstance woman in our culture particularly painful at this moment. Not all cultures are pronatalist – in Germany it is quite unknown and being childless or childfree is considered quite unremarkable, as is motherhood. However, this too has deep cultural roots, as the promotion of motherhood still carries a whiff of eugenics to the Germans.

A pronatalist culture is also, ironically, a hard one for mothers too, who are only able to share with each other and behind closed doors, the struggles and disappointments of their lives. In public, all they are 'allowed' to say is that motherhood is 'the most fulfilling thing I've ever done'.

I'm not saying that mothers are lying, but let's just say that in political terms they are perhaps being economical with the truth! Just as there is a cultural taboo about talking about childlessness, there's also a taboo about telling the truth about motherhood. It's as if there's a cultural magic spell currently assigned to Motherhood with a capital 'M' and mothers aren't allowed to break it.

> The fact is, life is harder than it looks in the glossy pages of magazines and modern motherhood isn't the picnic the adverts would have you believe.

It's for this reason that I think it's worth taking the time to deconstruct how many of the 'meanings' we've assigned to motherhood actually make sense, and whether hanging onto these ideas is doing us any favours. It may be time to refresh these thoughts as many of them are the products of the ideology of our times and not necessarily of our own thinking.

Ideology is that which everyone believes to be 'true', but it's actually a mixture of accepted prevalent beliefs that serve to support the dominant power group. Up until 500 years ago everyone thought the world was flat. That was an idea, not a truth and around it was created a powerful ideology of Western Europe being at 'the centre' of the world. So perhaps the 'belief' that a woman can only have a meaningful life if she is a mother may prove to be an ideological one and not the purely biological one that many of us have come to believe.

> After all, there was a time when women dreamt of lives other than that of mothers, precisely so that they could create lives of meaning.

It is the *meaning* we give to things, rather than the things themselves, that shapes our reality. And the meaning we give to things is something under our control, and can be changed.

HOW OUR CHILDHOODS COLOUR OUR FEELINGS ABOUT MOTHERHOOD

What messages did you pick up about motherhood when you were a child? In my case, I was an unplanned baby born to a teenage mother and the sudden burdens and limitations of motherhood were a struggle for her to adjust to. Having tasted the beginnings of freedom in the early 1960s, just a few years later she found herself 'respectably' and unhappily married, which was really the only choice for single mothers then unless you gave your baby up for adoption. And my mother made the incredibly brave decision not to.

Although I don't recall my mother ever telling me *not* to have children, she never actually encouraged me to have them either. Instead, she focused on all the amazing opportunities that awaited me as a child of the 1960s, the movement for women's equality and the pill. One of the 'messages' that I absorbed from this was that motherhood definitely wasn't the only option for women. It wasn't hard to see that she longed to leave the narrow domestic world of motherhood and get back the freedom and independence she'd tasted for a couple of years as a teenager; I could tell that she felt the bondage of her position as a dependent wife keenly. So, another message I picked up from this was 'to have a career and don't rely on a man'. Also, growing up with an unhappy mother and an aggressive stepfather, I unconsciously came to associate 'childhood' with fear and uncertainty, not love and safety. So, it was hardly surprising, I guess, that I was in no rush to start a family of my own.

But it's not just a challenging childhood that may have left you with complex unconscious or unexamined beliefs about motherhood. For those of us who grew up in a 'perfect' family, the chances are it was 'perfect' because your mother made it her life's work. And if you were an ambitious, bright girl you might have looked at what her life entailed and thought: *I'm not sure I could ever sacrifice myself the way she did.* You could see that she 'worked her fingers to the bone' on housework, gardening, baking, cleaning and worrying whilst seeming to have no life of her own outside of being your mother. You could see that she got no obvious status or recognition for what she did: 'Oh, I'm just a housewife', you may have heard her say, slightly apologetically, when asked. You may have never even heard people call her by her real name, but always as 'Mum' or 'So-and-So's Mother'. Whilst she may have encouraged you to have a broader life for yourself, you may have been unconsciously aware of the difficulties of trying to combine those aspirations with the kind of full-time, hands-on mothering you experienced and absorbed as the 'right way' to do it...

It's not just our own family environment that will have given us ideas about motherhood – there's the broader social environment we grew up in and the religious and cultural beliefs we absorbed as we grew into maturity. At my school, our sex education classes around the age of 16 consisted of it being drummed into our heads that getting pregnant was for 'losers' and that we'd be 'throwing away our lives' if we got pregnant. Looking back now, I can see that what our teachers were talking about were unplanned teenage pregnancies, but the message that I took, and from talking to other women I'm not alone in this, is that the hard thing is *not* getting pregnant, and that having a child ruins your life. For those of us who went on to have infertility problems or to sometimes feel that *not* having a child has 'ruined our life' this rings pretty hollow now.

Our current cultural fetishisation of motherhood was definitely not in place when I was a teenager, and the idea of our heroines getting pregnant and having babies was not something we wanted to know about or emulate. Debbie Harry having a baby? No way (she never did, by the way). Kate Bush having a baby? (She did, and disappeared from view.) It may not have been the same for everyone, but my peer group saw getting pregnant as a cop-out, uncool and somehow letting the side down.

However, I know other women who grew up during the same period whose families were more traditional and whose lives were focused around their faith and community. These intelligent and ambitious young women had to go *against* their family's expectations that they would marry young and have children in order to go to university and have a career. Their mothers wept and did all they could to persuade them to 'settle down' instead. It was seen as an either/or choice, not a both/and. In some ways those mothers were not as completely deluded as they seemed to us at the time. Sadly, it has certainly been the case for quite a few childless women that I've spoken with that their education and career have made it harder for them to find a partner in time to create a family. But still, none of them wished that they'd got married straight out of school and forgone their higher education.

If you were ambivalent about becoming a mother and hoped that 'life' would make that decision for you; that 'it would just happen one day' and then it didn't – it can be very painful to realise that some of that ambivalence came from your unexamined beliefs about childhood and motherhood. Finding this out 'too late' is incredibly painful and can often compound the sense of being a failure as a woman because you didn't even manage to get clear on how you *really* felt about having a family – something which we hear is meant to be an obvious and natural desire for women.

Quite often I talk with women around the age of 40 who've never wanted children and have been proudly childfree for a long time, but who are now wondering whether in fact they've made a mistake. They fear that maybe they do 'secretly' want a baby but that they just 'don't know it'. They fear waking up too late to their 'real' thoughts and feelings about having a family. So loaded and fraught has this seemingly 'obvious' and 'natural' decision become that there are now specialised 'Maybe Baby' coaches who work with women as they make this decision.

The fear of regret, of getting it wrong, seems to haunt many women as they come to the end of their fertility and aren't sure what to do, because it seems we now deem 'regret' to be the shameful punishment for not making the right decisions. It seems that we no longer fear that God will damn us, we fear damning ourselves.

Thinking that we are solely responsible for the outcome of our lives based on the quality of our own decisions can provoke an incredible level of anxiety. The philosopher Renata Salecl writes of this in her 2010 book 'Choice' when she describes an experience many of us will identify with, that of going into a supermarket and being overwhelmed and paralysed by the anxiety of choice. Her personal nemesis proves to be a cheese shop in Manhattan where she finds herself getting angrier and more irrational as her options expand when all she wanted was 'some cheese'.[21]

Choosing whether or not to be a mother is not one of those decisions you can take back to the shop, so the level of anxiety it can provoke can turn your life inside-out if you don't realise what's going on. Because there is absolutely no way to future-proof the decision to become, or not become, a mother. You can weigh up the pros and cons till the cows come home (and you'll find there are more cons than pros on a concrete level, which is why pronatalism exists, as well as the taboo of childlessness), but ultimately having a child is a leap of faith that you are committed to for the rest of your life. And if you get it wrong, you fear condemning yourself to a life of disabling regret. So, no pressure then!

EXERCISE 3: THE MEANINGS OF MOTHERHOOD

Grab a pile of Post-It notes (preferably in four different colours). Write each word or phrase that comes to mind in response to this exercise on a separate Post-It note (or separate small pieces of paper).

For each of the following prompts, write between five and ten responses to it on one colour of Post-It note. And then move on to the next prompt and the next colour. Don't think too hard about what you write. Just write the first things that come into your mind. It's not important at this stage that they 'make sense'.

- **1st Colour Post-It Note: 1st Prompt**
  One word or short phrase per note that springs to mind when you think of the word 'Mother'. Repeat 5-10 times.

- **2nd Colour Post-It Note: 2nd Prompt**
  One word or short phrase per note that springs to mind when you think of the word 'Children'. Repeat 5-10 times.

- **3rd Colour Post-It Note: 3rd Prompt**
  One word or short phrase per note about activities which you like 'doing' and which put you into a place of 'flow' (where time feels soft and passes in a flash). These might be activities that you feel are 'meaningful' to you in some way, or they might not be. Repeat 5-10 times.

- **4th Colour Post-It Note: 4th Prompt**
  One word or short phrase per note about ways of 'being' or 'feeling' that you enjoy (eg: calm, loving, laughing...) Repeat 5-10 times.

Arrange your responses in four vertical columns, with Prompt 1 as the furthest left column, and Prompt 4 as the last column on the right.

Now... step back, and take a look.

- Can you begin to see that some of the things, states, ways of feeling, etc that you have associated with motherhood and children (the first two columns) might actually be accessible through the activities you like doing (third column)?

- Can you see that some of the ways of being or feeling that bring you joy and meaning are actually open to you even without being a mother?

Choose one thing that you thought would only be accessible through motherhood (first and second columns) to do in the next week by doing an activity (third column) that brings meaning, joy and flow into your life (fourth column).

Commit to doing it this week. It doesn't have to be a big deal. If being in nature, sewing or writing feels meaningful and/or joyful to you, then do it. Often it's those things that have a 'creative' element to them that we resist the most. (We'll be looking more at why this might be in Chapter 10).

There's no right or wrong way to do this exercise – it's just a way to start loosening some of the fixed associations in your mind that you can *only* be happy, content and live a life that has meaning for you *if you are a mother.*

Now, undoubtedly, there are *some* aspects of being a mother that are irreplaceable – giving birth and the physical and emotional intimacy that passes between mother and child is not something we will ever experience. There are many things I will never experience in this lifetime, but that absolutely does not mean that I can't have a meaningful and fulfilling life without them.

REFLECTIONS ON THIS CHAPTER

In this chapter we've started to unpack some of the ideology surrounding motherhood in our culture and how we might have been influenced by it. Looking at this can be quite explosive so if you found yourself wanting to chuck this book across the room, I understand. Perhaps you thought 'I didn't buy this book so that you could run down motherhood!' which I didn't, by the way, but when our cherished beliefs are challenged, our first reaction is often to shoot the messenger.

It can be galling to realise that we've invested so much of our life force chasing a 'fantasy' version of motherhood. Even if we have sisters and friends with children and are privy to the day-to-day reality of their lives, those personal experiences still don't seem to counterbalance the vast weight of fantasy we are exposed to on a daily basis. Pronatalism is in the air we breathe; it takes a while to learn how to filter it out.

Reflecting on the messages we picked up in childhood can be a real eye-opener too and can bring up a lot of sadness and resentment. 'If only I'd known this earlier' is not an uncommon thought and a really tough one to digest.

If you did the 'Meanings of Motherhood' exercise you may have been surprised, relieved or baffled by it, but I hope it's helped you to begin to question some of your fixed beliefs; namely that not all of the things you believed were denied to you forever because of not having children are. If you committed to an activity you may have had to fight through a lot of resistance to actually do it! Strange as it may sound, our unhappiness may be an identity we've become used to. Beginning to break the shell of that identity can be very provocative and we may resist it fiercely.

Change is never easy, even when it's positive. For now, whatever you've done from this chapter, just know that by reading it you've already taken a big step and that your consciousness is shifting internally. The external changes will come when you feel ready. You can't force anyone else to change; and it's not that easy to force yourself to either. Time to try something different: kindness.

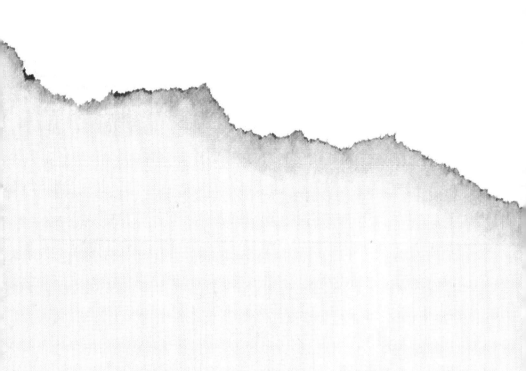

Grief is a dialogue **not**
a **monologue**.

CHAPTER 4

WORKING THROUGH THE GRIEF OF CHILDLESSNESS

THE TUNNEL

Many of us will probably remember a time when thinking about motherhood was something that dominated our waking and sleeping thoughts – when it was literally all we could think about. On the very first blog I wrote for Gateway Women in April 2011, I described this state of mind as 'the tunnel':

> *A narrow, cramped claustrophobic space that gets more cramped as each year passes. Made for one. The only view ahead is a very narrow shaft of light, somewhere off in the distance. And behind you in the dark is every wrong decision, every failed relationship, every missed opportunity.*

> *The tunnel. A lonely, pressurised space where you can't turn round, can't reverse, can't go sideways. And your only guides in this fetid space? The polarised opinions of others and your own, by now, thoroughly freaked-out self.*

Because, even though you may or may not have given the issue much thought, you've suddenly realised with an awful sickening thud that if you don't have a baby, you're not a real woman, you're on the shelf, you've failed.[22]

The tunnel is a place where we lose touch with reality and with ourselves as we become obsessed with the thought of having, or not having, a baby. It's what I've termed 'babymania'.

Some of us, myself included, can spend years in the tunnel, even decades. The experience is different for each of us but for me it was a sort of fugue state that I can only describe as a mixture of sleepwalking and panic. I lost some of the most precious years of my life whilst I was in the tunnel, made some terrible decisions and missed out on some fantastic opportunities. From talking to other women I know that my experience is something many of us can recognise, and which often only adds to our sense of shame and foolishness.

The reason the tunnel can have *such* a destructive effect on our health, morale, personality, career, ambition and peace of mind is that it's actually another way to describe the first stage of grief: denial.

GRIEF IS GOOD

In Western culture, we've become fairly hopeless at coping with grief, with loss. We fail to recognise its power, its meaning and its healing and run from it as if it were death itself. Yet grief is the emotional and psychological process that *enables* us to deal with loss. Avoiding it makes us emotional wrecks, unable to cope with life, unable to move forward.

Becoming aware of the possibility that we may not have children, that we may not have the family of our dreams, is a heartbreaking loss. Unlike many of the other losses we may have experienced, the end of fertility or the possibility of bearing a biological child is an irrevocable and definite loss. It's a kind of psychological death and it's profound. Facing up to it changes us forever.

What we, and others, often fail to realise is the depth and reach of our loss: that not only will we never have children but we will never have a family. We will never watch them grow up, never throw children's birthday parties, never get a chance to heal the wounds of our own childhood by doing things differently with *our* children. We'll never be grandmothers and never give the gift of grandchildren to our parents. We'll never be the mother of our partner's children and hold that precious place in their heart. We'll never stand shoulder-to-shoulder with our siblings and watch our children play together. We'll never be part of the community of mothers, never be considered a 'real' woman. And when we die, there is no one to take our lifetime's learnings onto the next generation.

If you take the time to think about it all in one go, which is more than most of us are ever likely to do because of the breathtaking amount of pain involved, it's a testament to our strength that we're still standing at all.

And yet, because the loss of our future children is an *invisible* loss, we often fail to recognise *ourselves* that what we are experiencing is grief, and others don't seem to have a clue what depth of pain and distress we are in. Some women are in such pain that they find themselves having suicidal fantasies. I did. It's not that I wanted to die, I just didn't want to live the rest of my life with this level of pain.

If we miscarry, fail to conceive or never have the opportunity to try for a baby, our loss remains invisible and unrecognised by others. And, because our loss isn't recognised and reflected back to us with kindness and empathy, we often give up seeking understanding from others and may instead learn to block our pain with all kinds of self-medication including drinking too much, overeating, overworking or becoming a sort of recluse. Doing so, we may remain stuck in a quagmire of unprocessed grief for years.

If we had lost a living family by some tragic event, we would never expect ourselves to 'get over it' completely. Yet we, and others, expect those of us who are childless-by-circumstance to pick ourselves up, dust ourselves off, count our blessings and get on with things. No wonder so many of us are struggling. The treatment we currently receive is not just neglectful, it's downright cruel. And sadly, knowing no better, many of us treat ourselves in exactly the same way.

> Grief heals us, but we cannot do it alone. We cannot 'wait it out'. Time does not heal: grieving heals. But it cannot heal until it is witnessed and held jointly, with great tenderness, in the heart and soul of another. Just like love.

Grief is a dialogue, not a monologue. And until we find a place to have that dialogue, it stays wedged in our hearts like a splinter. And it festers as it waits, infecting our life and our souls with sadness. It is vital that as childless women we grieve our losses and in doing so, allow that grief to heal our hearts. Without grieving, we're stuck fast. And without empathetic company with whom to do our grief work, we can stay stuck fast for a very long time indeed.

Miracle Baby Stories

One of the ways that the culture colludes with us in our denial is with what I call the 'miracle baby story'. This is the fairly predictable response we often get from others when the conversation strays into the fact that we don't have children, and never will.

The media features regular 'miracle baby stories' of women who despaired for years about their childlessness and then had a baby after their nth round of IVF, through egg-donation, surrogacy, etc. Or sensationalist stories of women in their 50s conceiving naturally, or women in their 60s and even 70s having a babies using donor eggs. There is even a whole Wikipedia page[23] devoted to these extraordinary feats of human reproduction with data about the woman's age, father's sperm, reproductive technologies involved and live births resulting.

When someone says to us, 'But you mustn't give up hope! I read about this woman who…' it's helpful to recall (and perhaps even to gently point out) that the reason these stories are in the media in the first place is because they are *news*. They are not the norm and they are referred to as 'miracles' because they are *rare*. Offering a childless woman this kind of 'hope' is akin to suggesting to someone with financial problems that they're going to win the lottery. And for every woman who makes the news or gets onto that Wikipedia page, how many other heartbreaking stories must there be of the women and couples who devastated their bodies, bank balances, relationships, careers and mental health chasing a miracle baby only to end up without one? Their stories are never told because they're not news, but they are just as much part of the story.

Just as *we* have difficulty accepting and processing our loss, so do others. As I've said, we've become culturally spooked by grief, by loss. It runs counter to the message of consumerism and science that anything can be fixed if you're smart enough, make good decisions, have enough data and throw enough money at it.

Whether we realise it consciously or not we humans, to a greater or lesser degree, feel each other's emotions – the mirror neurons in our brain fire when we see someone experiencing an emotion so that we feel the same. And so when others trot out miracle baby stories to our face, what they are doing is using those stories as an unconscious shield to stop us feeling *our* pain so they can stop feeling what it triggers in them – *their* ungrieved losses. After all, we all carry so many. They may not realise what they are doing but by defending themselves in that moment they deny us the one thing we need to heal: understanding, recognition, empathy. Even just, 'I'm so sorry, that must be hard some days' would be a rare balm to our bruised souls.

> Luckily, grief is patient, persistent and wise. It will keep seeking out that empathetic 'other' until your healing can be completed. Grief is not out to hurt you, it longs to heal you.

Not that long ago a Gateway Woman posed a hypothetical question to me – she wondered what I would do if I were to meet a new partner and he wanted to try for a baby; would I be willing to go through IVF with a donor egg? This was not something I'd ever considered before.

'No', I said, without hesitation.

'Wow, that seems pretty clear!' she said, 'How can you be so sure?'

I was pretty surprised myself but heard myself replying, 'Because I don't want to have a baby at this age. That time of my life has passed. I'm no longer looking to become a mother, that's over. I'm in a new phase of my life now. I've moved on.'

Grief had healed what was once a wound into a scar. And I can live with a scar, move forward with a scar. It will always be a tender spot, but it's no longer a festering wound.

Not having children broke my heart, no doubt about it. But grief healed it bigger. I am a different person, a bigger person for having grieved the family I longed for. I will never 'get over' not having a family (it's not the flu), but that doesn't mean that I can't build a new life. There are moments when something touches the scar on my heart, and I won't lie, it can feel like being kicked in the chest. But these days I've learned that rather than contract against the pain, I literally open myself to it – pushing my shoulders back, imagining opening my heart and I breathe in the pain, letting it flow through me and out of me. *More healing* I say to myself, *another corner of my heart healing*.

The things that trigger these moments are totally unpredictable. It can be the shining hair of a child in the street as they turn their head, or a look that passes between a mother and her child. It can also be something that seemingly has nothing to do with children. For example, very recently a houseguest dropped a heavy saucepan onto my most precious set of china, a set of six plates that had been given to me as wedding present by my maid of honour and my oldest friend from school. The plates had survived intact in storage for ten years and had only just been unpacked now that I had a home again. My guest was incredibly sorry and offered to replace the china, which I accepted, even though I knew that the set was a limited edition and irreplaceable – I just couldn't bring myself to tell him that just yet. I walked away and went into the bathroom, feeling the loss keenly and wanting to wail with pain, yet also not wanting to upset him any further – after all, accidents happen. As I sat in the bathroom I thought of those plates, of the dear friend who had bought them for me, of meeting her when I moved to a new school at 15, of her sleeping in the bed next to me the night before my wedding. And then I thought: *what will happen to my china when I die? I've got no one to give it to.* It was an awful moment, but then I realised that once I was gone, they'd just be plates. Nothing more, just plates. I realised that it was all just 'stuff' and that what was important about them were my memories and that *they* were still intact. I came out of the bathroom and told my guest not to worry about replacing them. 'They're just plates', I said, 'accidents happen'. In the past, something like this would have had me in bits for a week – the visceral realisation that I have no descendants, no one to whom anything of mine will mean anything. However, having done my grief work such moments still hurt but, at a deeper level, I understand that I'm OK and that I can handle it. My reality no longer scares me, although sometimes, like on this occasion, it shocks me when I become aware of a new aspect of my loss.

Grandchildren Grief

You'd think that once you'd grieved the loss of the family you'd longed for and found a way to move on with your life, you'd be sorted; that you'd be able to deal with any baby-related issue without it flooring you, ever again. Or at least without it making you run to the bathroom for a cry at family events or at work.

But no, that's not how it works, sorry. As I mentioned before, grief leaves a scar and a scar will always be a tender spot. And when something touches it, it reminds you of your loss.

However, if by the time other people's grandchildren start appearing, you haven't had a chance to do your grief work, but instead found a way to push it under the surface and move on as best you could at the time, you may find that you are unexpectedly thrown back into a pit of despair. Not having grandchildren may bring back the pain of not having been a mother, and friends that you may have reconnected with once their children had left home once again start becoming less available.

I had a hint of what's to come a few years ago when my teenage goddaughter walked up to me with a mutual-friend's baby on her hip and said, 'I can't wait till I have my own baby!' With a sickening lurch I realised that *it was all going to start happening again one day soon* – watching everyone but me have grandchildren. The vision of this beautiful young woman at the very beginning of her childbearing years walking towards me with a baby on her hip was so archetypal, so full of promise and joy, and yet so coloured by my own loss. A bittersweet tear popped out of the corner of my eye and joined my genuine delight in her excitement, as well as my fervent hopes that *her* dreams of a family come true for her. *May she never know the taste of these tears*, I prayed.

I'm in a better place now and recently met my new godson and found I was able to enjoy spending time cuddling, feeding and getting to know a 3-month-old baby – something I couldn't have coped with a couple of years ago. Doing our grief work, rather than living with unprocessed grief, really does heal our hearts.

Many older childless women have been in touch with me to share how 'left out' they feel because they don't have grandchildren. Coming from a generation where opportunities *other* than becoming a mother were more limited, they suffer in silence. For most of them there has been no opportunity to grieve the loss of the family they wanted; coming from a more buttoned-up era emotionally, they tell me they just 'got on with things'. But now they find they're really struggling over the grandchildren issue.

> Think about it for a moment: how many empowering and happy images can you find in the media of women or couples over 60 that don't include grandchildren somewhere in the picture?

Many women in their 60s and older didn't have access to the kind of reproductive medicine we have today – the first successful 'test tube baby', Louise Brown, was born in 1978.[24] This meant that they were forced to come to terms with their loss as something irrevocable much sooner than many younger women. In some ways, this might be seen as a blessing as the endless hope of today's fertility treatments can prove to be a problem in itself. I've written of hope as being the most toxic fertility drug of all and it's touched a chord with many women who've been through the fertility mill and come out the other end with nothing but huge debt and a broken heart.

Depending on where you are with your grief over your childlessness you're going to react differently to being 'the odd one out' again when grandchildren come around. Like I've said, you can't 'wait out' grief.

Although it may not feel like it's got anything going for it at all, the pain that comes up around grandchildren is actually signalling another opportunity for the loving energy of grief to heal you. And these days, thanks to the internet, there's a greater chance that you can reach out to others who'll understand and support you as you do your grief work. Your grief over not having grandchildren is a gift from the family you never had. If you choose to unwrap this precious gift in the presence of others who understand, you'll finally be able to find a safe home in your heart for that loss and begin the next act of your life as a powerful, happy and integrated older woman.

Reach out to other women who are dealing with grandchildren grief through a growing number of online networks (see Appendix for more details) and you'll find others ready to unwrap that gift with you. And once you've done that you can celebrate the life you've got and enjoy your friends' stories of their grandchildren without losing the plot. Well that's the plan anyway. I'm afraid completing your grieving will not inoculate you against boredom or irritation!

THE FIVE STAGES OF GRIEF MODEL

The Five Stages of Grief model was developed by Elisabeth Kübler-Ross[25] as a hypothesis from her work with terminally ill patients and was set out in her 1969 book 'On Death and Dying'. Although it has often been contested, it has not been bettered and has been hugely influential in the West in helping us to understand the power, process and necessity of grief in dealing with loss.

Sometimes, Kübler-Ross's model is referred to as 'DABDA' which is an acronym for the names of the five stages:

1. **D**enial

2. **A**nger

3. **B**argaining

4. **D**epression

5. **A**cceptance.

GRIEF IS A SPIRAL

The linear, list-like nature of Kübler-Ross's model can give the impression that grief is a tidy process, one that moves cleanly and clearly from one stage to the next, but there are many who prefer to visualise it as something slightly more organic; as a spiral. Kübler-Ross recognised this herself, commenting later that 'the stages are not linear. People do not necessarily go through all of them.'[26]

A spiral has a trajectory, but one which curves and dips back on itself, as does grief. I also think that different parts of our experience are in different positions on the spiral – we are not completely 'in denial' about everything related to our loss and whilst we might be aware of the fact that we will never have a child, we can still be thrown back into 'depression' or 'anger' by the realisation that we will never have grandchildren.

Grief is a powerful, life-changing human emotional process, like love. Indeed, another Elizabeth, Queen Elizabeth II, said that 'grief is the price we pay for love'.[27] But I have a different view.

> I have come to believe that grief is actually the *gift* of love. We cannot grieve that which we have not loved; and we cannot be healed from the loss of that love without grief.

Grief is not about 'getting over' something, but about healing around it until that loss is integrated into our new identity. The tears of grief are not a sign of weakness but of healing.

So, whilst the Kübler-Ross model gives us a framework to understand grief and a shared language to use as we support each other in our grief work, we need to realise that grief remains an experience as subjective for each of us as love is.

If we think of grief as a form of love, rather than a set of steps to arrive at a destination, it becomes easier to understand that it is ever changing, often surprising, deeply revealing and not always convenient. Transformation is never straightforward.

Denial: The First of the Five Stages of Grief

We can only be aware of those things that we are no longer in denial about or which we are in the process of coming out of denial about. There will always be some things we are still in denial about; it's called being human. Melody Beattie describes denial as a duvet that we pull over our heads to protect us from a painful awareness and which gradually, as the conditions around us feel safer, we pull down, bit by bit.[28] I like the gentleness of picturing it as warm and cosy protection, rather than something we're doing wrong by avoiding thinking about it.

There's nothing wrong with denial, despite the way it's bandied about in popular parlance; it's a very wise psychological mechanism that protects us from anguish we're not yet ready to deal with.

> Without denial to protect us, if we were to feel the full force of our losses in one go, rather than gradually, the shock might well be unendurable.

Perhaps continuing with infertility treatments long after we could afford to, either financially or emotionally, is a form of denial. Or being unshakably convinced that we would have one of those 'miracle babies' – after all, that's what everyone keeps telling us. It may be as simple as chopping a few years off our age or as complex as allowing someone to presume that a niece or nephew is our own child without correcting their mistake.

You might realise that when you used to convince yourself that having periods meant you were still fertile you were in denial about the quality of your remaining eggs. Or perhaps you used to scour the media for any stories about women your age having children and keep those articles like talismans. I had one in the bottom of my jewellery box for years. Or then again, perhaps you let people think you were 'still trying' long after you and your partner had stopped fertility treatments.

In 12-Step recovery programmes (like Alcoholics Anonymous), denial is often explained by the acronym **D**on't **E**ven k**N**ow **I A**m **L**ying. There is a lot of truth in this (no pun intended!) because denial is impervious to logic or reality. It protects us completely. You might even recall that before you fully acknowledged that you were never going to become a mother someone tried to discuss it with you, perhaps even to offer you some support, and you brushed them off slightly aggressively as having got your situation 'completely wrong'. That's denial.

ANGER: THE SECOND OF THE FIVE STAGES OF GRIEF

When we resent the fact that 'she' got a family but we didn't. When we find ourselves saying unkind things about 'mothers'. When we feel bitter, judgemental and outraged by the way we are treated by society as childless women, what we're experiencing is anger.

> There's nothing wrong with anger, despite its bad reputation. Like all human emotions, it's there for a reason – it's a response to injustice. It's a protection mechanism.

However, we need to be wise in understanding the difference between healthy anger and unhealthy anger. Healthy anger is a motivating force that gives us the energy to make changes in our life. Unhealthy anger shows up as resentfulness, bitterness, envy and a toxic negativity that can form a shield that keeps everyone at a safe distance. I've met childless women so angry that it's very hard to be in their presence at all – and often what they are angriest about (and blame everyone else for) is their isolation…

Some of the anger we feel about how overlooked we are as women because we don't have children is what I would think of as justified anger. It encourages us to change the way things are. It doesn't give us the right to berate anyone, but it does give us the nerve to stand up for ourselves and for others who are not yet ready to do so.

Bitterness, spiteful remarks, bitching, envy and jealousy may be signs that we are stuck in grief-related anger about our childlessness. Those feelings *will* pass as we move through our grief but they can reappear when we come face-to-face with a new version of an old situation – like an ex-partner having a baby or grandchild or even just a TV advert showing a multi-generational family including children and grandchildren.

Anger is a very potent emotion both emotionally and physically. It stimulates our fight-flight-freeze response and fills our system with powerful chemicals that can result in stress-related illness and erratic behaviour if not dispersed through physical activity or an emotional release of some kind. Whilst punching a pillow doesn't work for everyone, going for a run or, one of my favourites, deep-cleaning the bathroom, can really help to disperse the biochemicals produced as part of the anger response. Some kind of creative practice like painting, singing or gardening can be a helpful release too – I find writing to try and correct or respond to injustice allows me some resolution. After all, that's how Gateway Women began.

Anger doesn't always look or sound angry. Some women, brought up in families and cultures where girls weren't 'allowed' to be angry turn it on themselves instead and overeat, drink and develop a supercritical inner voice that makes everything they do 'wrong'. An inner bitch can be as toxic, if not more so, as an outer one.

Alternatively, some of us may have learned to use anger as a way to suppress or hide our vulnerability when we were very young and know just how to use it to protect ourselves. In that case, grief may turn our anger-dial right up to ten and we may be furious with absolutely everyone and everything. White-hot fury at the world is understandable but it's a scorched-earth policy and you may lose jobs, partners, friends and the support of your family if you don't realise soon enough that anger is burning up your life. Anger management classes aren't going to help: you need to do your grief work.

Anger can show up in all kinds of ways: the 'flight' response may show up with you running a marathon or single-handedly landscaping the garden. Anger makes things happen, so you may change careers, leave your partner and move country whilst under its galvanising influence, only to wake up one day and wonder what the hell happened! The 'fight' response often manifests in argumentative, unreasonable, fault-finding intolerance towards yourself and others and destructive behaviour. The 'freeze' response (playing dead in mammals) can include emotional paralysis, staying in a toxic relationship, an inability to make decisions and a loss of libido, but may also show up in withdrawal (getting away) behaviours such as substance abuse, overwork or obsessive TV or internet use – anything that 'zones us out'.

Despite all this, and although we may not realise it – anger is a loyal friend. It may not be nice or pretty, but it's a hell of an *activating* emotion. Anger is the fire of life, the fire in the belly. It makes stuff happen if you let it. Using it wisely can take a lifetime; suppressing it is an illusion – it just goes underground and it'll come up somewhere else.

BARGAINING: THE THIRD OF THE FIVE STAGES OF GRIEF

Bargaining is a strange state and a hard one to pin down sometimes. It involves negotiating with reality, or 'magical thinking' as a way of trying to make our loss go away.

Whilst there is still hope of having a baby, bargaining tends to take the form of things we could change in order to make it more likely that we will have a child. It might be that we think that if we're 'a better person' we'll get pregnant, or we think of ways we could behave that might make us 'deserve' to win the lottery and be able to afford to have a baby on our own or pay for more fertility treatments. We might return to a faith of our youth or develop obsessions or superstitions.

However, once we are *sure* that we are no longer able to have a biological child, bargaining takes more subtle forms. We might decide that if we 'stop this' or 'start that', we'll meet a partner with children. It's also not uncommon to fantasise about friends or siblings being killed suddenly so that we become guardians of their children. These thoughts are normal, even though they shock us with their ghoulishness.

We may also enter a phase of compulsively counting our blessings as a way of 'warding off' our grief over childlessness. This has a different flavour from genuine gratitude and can be heard in thoughts like,

'I wouldn't have been able to do *this* if I'd had children,' when we're travelling or, 'Thank goodness I didn't have a child' when something bad happens like a relationship breakdown, job loss or chronic illness. We may even try to convince ourselves that we didn't *really* want children, but rather that we were just going along with social conventions, with what was expected of us.

> What's happening is that we're trying to weigh our loss against life and decide that it's OK. But it's not. If it were, it wouldn't be the first thing that sprang to mind when our life took a new turn.

It's as if we are still holding a space in our life psychically for that child. We aren't letting go, not completely, not yet.

We may even fantasise about some kind of Faustian pact whereby we make a sacrificial deal with a higher power in order for the chance to become a mother. It's not logical, but it's the way we work through all the possible, and impossible, ways we might try to avoid our loss before we are ready to face and accept it.

DEPRESSION: THE FOURTH OF THE FIVE STAGES OF GRIEF

Withdrawing from the world to lick our wounds is a natural part of adjusting to loss. It's the time when we give up hope and face what's underneath all our denial, anger and bargaining – the reality of what we've lost: the loss itself.

Being depressed is not necessarily always a problem – it has a valuable part to play in giving us the rest and space we need to reconstruct our identity after losing someone or something very dear to us. It's a natural response. However, when it moves from a deep sadness into a clinical depression that does not lift, it's important to see a doctor. One of the symptoms of clinical depression can be that *you* don't realise you're depressed – so if others close to you suggest that you are and yet you hadn't thought so, it might be a good idea to get it checked out.

> The depression that is a part of grief will pass when it has given you the space, rest and introspection you need to move forward with your healing journey.

Some typical thoughts I've heard from women in the depression stage of the grief cycle are, 'What's the point of anything any more… I'm never going to be a mother.' These thoughts and trying to find a way to resolve them can form cyclical and repetitive patterns of thinking that go literally round and round until we are mentally exhausted and distressed. In fact, depression used to be called 'mental exhaustion'.

Sometimes, we may withdraw from our partner and from sexual intimacy because it seems pointless if there is no hope of a baby resulting from the act of love. We may push our partners away, trying to make them leave us because we have 'failed them'. We might stop taking care of ourselves physically, not being bothered to make an effort with the way we look, or staying fit. We may feel de-sexed as women now that we will never be 'real women'. We may wonder what the point of us is as women if we are never to be mothers.

There may also be fear and anxiety in the depression stage as we begin to contemplate the rest of our lives without children, of growing old and dying without children to care for us. We may fear that our partner will leave us, or that we will never meet someone and will be alone and miserable for the rest of our lives. (We'll be looking at ways to think differently about these fears in Chapter 12.)

We may cry and mourn in the stereotypical sense; feeling regretful, unable to see, engage with, or in some cases even *look* at children because our pain is so acute. We may find that it seems we are suddenly surrounded by children, by pregnant women, by grandchildren and that withdrawing from the world seems to be the only way to cope. We have no energy, our sleep patterns change (insomnia or sleeping much more than usual) and our appetite changes too (usually a loss of appetite, but sometimes eating a lot of comfort food).

We reject those who try to cheer us up and can be quite aggressive towards them if they persist; we are in a deeper place than that, and we know that's where we need to be.

Acceptance: The Fifth of the Five Stages of Grief

Ah, acceptance. Sounds nice, doesn't it…

In reality it's a mixed bag. Because what it means is accepting fully and completely right down to our very bones that we will never have children, never be mothers, never be grandmothers. That the millions of years of genetic feats of survival that created us stop here. That when we die, we die more absolutely than someone who knows that they 'live on' in their children.

> Acceptance is about coming to terms with our destiny and making peace with it. It doesn't mean we like it, or that we think it's fair. It just is what it is.

It doesn't mean that we won't be sad about how things have worked out but rather that we are no longer hopeful of any other outcome and so we stop fighting it. We accept it.

Acceptance does not mean that we go quietly. But what it *does* mean is that the energy that was locked up in our grief becomes available to us again, to dedicate towards a new future. Our past, and all the wrong turns, twists of fate, decisions made when five years old and left unexamined, biological complications, timing misses and misunderstandings that led to our childlessness become less important. We stop raking over them, we forgive ourselves (and others) involved in the drama, and we move on. We start thinking about what's next, rather than what might have been.

Grief heals. What was an open wound is now a scar. And we are ready to face life again, on its terms, not ours. We are ready to start thinking about our Plan B.

What is Grief Work?

Grief is passive; grieving is active. The good news is that once you begin your grief work you'll find that grief *isn't* a life-sentence of misery, but that it can start 'moving' quite quickly. This can also be slightly bewildering and may bring up feelings of guilt. I still sometimes get pangs of guilt that I'm out the other side of my grieving – it's quite natural and is called 'survivor's guilt'. The thought that goes with it for me is: *Well, if I've managed to get past my grief, that probably means I didn't really want to be a mother!* I know that's not true, I know how I suffered and how much I lost during those years of longing. But there's a little part of me that still craves the identity of the lost and grief-stricken woman I was. But then I remind myself that grief is an *emotional* process, not a *logical* one. It's about healing my heart so that life makes sense again, although sometimes the process itself seems to make little sense!

> Grief work is simply finding a way to process your grief with others who totally 'get it'.

Here are some ideas for doing your grief work, but this is by no means an exhaustive list:

- Seeing a grief counsellor or therapist – you might want to ask if they have experience with childlessness-related grief as many of us have found that therapists are not immune to the same unconscious prejudices as the rest of society. It's important too that you feel you 'click' with them when you first meet them - if you don't, keep looking and trust your first impressions. The quality of the relationship has a big impact on your experience as this is an *intimate relationship* you're entering, albeit a professional one.

- Doing some form of creative practice to produce work inspired by your loss and in a nurturing collective way where you can share that with others. It might be creative writing, music, singing, sculpture, painting, etc. If such a group doesn't exist in your area, you might like to think about approaching a grief counsellor and asking them to start one, or starting your own with a group of other childless-by-circumstance women.

- Attending a workshop or group for childless-by-circumstance women.

- Taking an *active* part in an online community for childless-by-circumstance women such as the Gateway Women Online Community (see Appendix).

- Taking an *active* part in an online grief community such Melody Beattie's 'Grief Club' (see Appendix).

- Setting up a Gateway Women Group, Reading Group or Meetup in your area (see Appendix).

- Writing a blog about your grief, or commenting on other grief-related blogs in order to get a dialogue going. This can be anonymous – whatever makes it possible for you to share your experience with others who understand and respond.

- Buddying-up with another childless-by-circumstance woman and working through this book together – you can connect through online communities at first and then progress to meeting up face-to-face.

- Reading books about grief and discussing them with other childless-by-circumstance women either online or face-to-face. (See Appendix for recommended reading).

- Becoming familiar with Kübler-Ross's Five Stages of Grief as they show up in all areas of life. Learning to name what you are experiencing with increasing precision will really help you process your grief.

- Doing the 'Declutter Your Dreams' exercise (at the end of Chapter 7).

- Talking, talking, talking about your situation with other women who 'get it' until you're bored of talking about it. Boredom with talking about our story is a good sign that we've processed that part of our grief. Usually, our story 'shifts' at this point and we start to look at it in a different way. This is what's called 'processing' our grief. It's an ongoing process though… each layer needs to be processed. I'm not sure it ever stops, but it certainly gets less painful the more we process it.

- Listening, listening, listening to other childless-by-circumstance women and being that non-judgemental, advice-free and empathetic sounding-board that we all need to do our grief work.

- Learning to be kind to yourself during grief – it can be exhausting.

> Grieving is as individual as loving – so there may be ways that work for you that I haven't listed. If it allows you to communicate your experience and feel heard and understood in a non-judgemental and empathetic way – if perhaps it makes you cry healing tears that leave you feeling better not worse – then it's grief work.

EXERCISE 4: DOING YOUR GRIEF WORK

Look back over each of Kübler-Ross's Five Stages of Grief in this chapter and write down how you have experienced, or are experiencing, each stage.

Keep this with you over the next week and see if you can add to it as you become more aware of the different stages of grief and how they are showing up for you. Be gentle with yourself and don't worry if you're not sure 'where' you are in the grief process. Just becoming aware that you are grieving may be all you need for things to start shifting.

This is not a test. It's about becoming a gentle witness to your own grief, so that you can work out what you need to do, and what support you'd like to get right now to continue your grief work.

REFLECTIONS ON THIS CHAPTER

In this chapter, we've started exploring how grief over our childlessness has affected us and how it continues to do so. Depending on how much grief work you've done, this may all be new to you, or you may be relieved to discover that you're further along in the process than you realised.

However, living as we do in a culture that is in denial about grief and loss and which does not recognise our loss at all, we may find that not only do we have more grief work to do, but that by allowing ourselves to grieve our childlessness, other ungrieved losses start surfacing too. It might be the dog that died when you were six or how you felt when your parents divorced. Each of us has a history of loss and if it's come up for healing, try not to push it down again.

If the losses that begin to surface are deep losses from childhood, like the death of a parent or another major trauma, you may want to think about seeking the help of a bereavement or trauma therapist. Try not to panic about this because if the grief is coming up now then it is ready to heal you and you are ready to allow it. However, like all grief work, you cannot do it alone. This is not about you being too weak to deal with it, it's just that that's not how grief works – it needs understanding company. You may find that seeking the support of other childless-by-circumstance women is enough, or you may wish to supplement that with other support. Trust yourself and the grief process. Grief is kind and gentle, but we can be rough and mean to ourselves. Grief wants to heal you, not hurt you.

If you did the 'Doing Your Grief Work' exercise, how did you find it? Often women in my groups and workshops find learning about the Kübler-Ross 'Five Stages of Grief' model a great help and having a way to 'name' their feelings hugely relieving. 'I just thought I was going crazy', is a not-uncommon response. Also, many of them (myself included) didn't know that what they were experiencing was grief. It's a good idea to re-read Chapter 4 whenever you get stuck and take an action using some of the suggestions in 'What is Grief Work' to obtain some relief and move forward. Learning to proactively work with grief rather than waiting for it to pass is a habit that will reap dividends for the rest of your life.

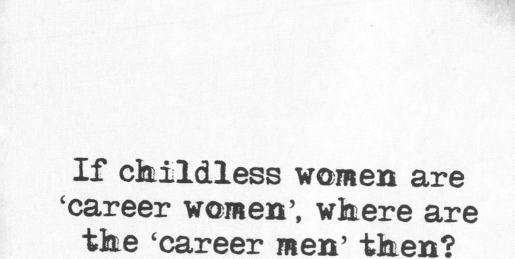

If childless women are
'career women', where are
the 'career men' then?

CHAPTER 5

LIBERATING YOURSELF FROM THE OPINIONS OF OTHERS

So, Have You Got Kids Then?

Once upon a time, if we went to the hairdresser's we'd be asked an innocuous social question such as, 'Been anywhere nice on holiday?' But these days, whether it's at the hairdresser, the bikini-waxing parlour, the dentist, a business conference or a party, the question often seems to be, 'So, have you got kids then?' or perhaps, 'So, how old are yours then?'

No doubt you've got your own horror story about being quizzed in public but I think the most hurtful one I ever experienced was whilst at my father-in-law's funeral with my soon to be ex-husband who was out of rehab for the occasion. An elderly woman collared me to tell me 'how selfish' my generation were, 'too obsessed with their careers to have children.' The truth was that at this point, my husband and I had been trying to conceive for about nine years, and I'd never even met or spoken to this woman before. I still have no idea who she was. It was already a very upsetting day and she managed to make it 100% worse. I'm sure you've got a few of these stinging and hurtful remarks lodged in your heart forever too.

It's also really tough when people presume that I *do* have children, but that they're just not here at the moment. 'Isn't it great when they go back to school?' a woman might say to me at the beginning of the new school term in a supermarket checkout. Or, when it's presumed that we *chose* not to have them, 'Such a good idea not having kids – wish I'd thought of that!'

I do understand that it's hard on men who wanted to be fathers too, but it seems that they are not exposed to these comments with the same relentless frequency as women are. And although an older man without children may be viewed with a certain suspicion as some kind of potential child molester, which is not something women have to cope with, often it is presumed that they just don't have children *yet*. Male factor infertility, being childless by relationship or any of the many other reasons that might be involved in a man's childlessness are rarely considered. Nor does it seem to occur to most that involuntary childlessness might be a source of great pain and grief for men too.

However, if we put ourselves for a moment in the shoes of our unsuspecting inquisitors, they can't win, no matter what they say.

If they know it's a delicate area and avoid it like the plague, we feel left out. If they *do* go there, on some days we're quite likely to go ashen-faced and leave the room, whilst at other times we're happy to look at their children's photos. We might rail at them for their thoughtlessness or harangue them for not inviting us to their kids' parties. But more often than not, there'll just be an awkward silence and they'll find someone 'easier' to talk to. And once again we'll be left with the sense that there's something 'wrong' with us, that we 'don't fit' and that perhaps the most socially convenient thing we could do would be to crawl under a rock and stay there. I call these the 'tumbleweed moments' and learning to cope with them is a big part of dealing with the unwanted identity of 'that childless woman'.

There was a time when I would dread the moment when someone would lob a 'Do you have kids' hand-grenade in my direction, but these days I see it as a kind of litmus test, a way of finding out exactly where I am on the pH scale between 'Totally OK with it' and 'So gutted I could punch you'. And, to be honest, it varies, although mostly these days I just find myself marvelling at their utter social cluelessness that trying to talk to a woman without children is beyond their repertoire: *We all used to be childless once, think; it's not that hard!*

Some days I'm thrilled to arrive home to a quiet house with just the cat to feed and other times I simply can't quite believe that this is how my life turned out. Just as when I was a teenager at school, getting 'up-the-duff' or 'in the club' (as we charmingly called it) was something that happened to 'other girls', being a divorced and childless middle-aged woman was an identity nothing prepared me for. Thinking about growing old without my soulmate and without the family I thought we would have sometimes surprises me so much it temporarily knocks the wind out of me.

> All of us childless-by-circumstance women are accidental pioneers. We didn't choose this difference, this role.

But these days, instead of thinking, 'Why me?' I think, 'Why not me?' I'm not special or different from any other woman and this is just the way the dice rolled. It could be much worse. But it varies from day to day. On bad days my grief over never being a mother, never being a grandmother, never being the mother of my partner's children, never being a part of the community of mothers, never being an accepted and valued member of society... well, it sucks so badly that I have to have a lie down till I get my nerve back. But such 'griefy days', as I call them, are getting rarer.

It's hard for others to realise (or believe) what an effort of will, self-belief and courage it takes to be a proud and well-adjusted childless-by-circumstance woman in our culture today. Because, in fact, no one's all that bothered about how life turns out for us. As long as we pay our taxes, don't complain about the injustices and prejudices we face, tolerate endless stories about other people's families and stick around to look after our elderly parents, our presence is tolerated. But I want more than being 'tolerated' and I'm pretty sure you do too!

THE TABOO OF CHILDLESSNESS

There is no 'acceptable' way to talk about childlessness, either voluntary or involuntary. It's a taboo and like all taboos, the way it's policed is that talking about it is seen as shameful and embarrassing. No one wants to risk raising the subject with us in case they embarrass us (a mild form of shame) or we embarrass them. Childless women stay silent on the subject, even with other women who don't have children, 'just in case'. Many women I work with in Gateway Women workshops and groups have a childless aunt or relative, but when I suggest to them that they talk to them about it, you'd think I'd asked them to commit a crime! They usually don't know her story, just some family whispers. Often they presume she chose to be childless, but when I ask if they are sure, they realise that this might just be the accepted family narrative.

> Nobody talks about childlessness so it's never a topic of conversation. And the longer this emotional policing continues, the more shame attaches itself to the subject of childlessness and it becomes even harder to talk about. That's how taboos work.

It only takes two people to start breaking a taboo: one to talk about it and another one to listen and be changed by that conversation. For some reason, I am one of the women in our generation who has chosen to break this taboo, and I'm liberating others by doing so. It's a bit like

'The Emperor's New Clothes' – the story where the child points out the 'truth' (that the emperor is naked) and this allows everyone else to admit what they knew all along but didn't dare speak.

Homosexuality was described at Oscar Wilde's trial as 'The love that dare not speak its name'[29] and, in some ways, I think 'coming out' as childless or childfree carries a similar stigma. I'm sure that our friends, family and society would be horrified to know that this is how we feel and would deny it vociferously, but until they've walked a day in our shoes, it's hard to 'see' the taboo. It's culturally invisible. Hopefully not for much longer though. It has only taken a generation to see some really positive change in attitudes towards homosexuality and I hope that we can do the same for childlessness. We just need to stick together and stop believing that mainstream opinion is any kind of 'truth'.

One of my dearest friends (who is a mother) came to a public talk I gave to a group of Gateway Women on International Women's Day in March 2012. She was there to support me personally as it was the largest public talk I'd given at that point, but what struck her the most was the way the women in the audience behaved. A childless-by-circumstance documentary filmmaker wanted to film my talk, but none of the women in the audience was prepared to be seen on camera (even the backs of their heads). They were too scared that someone they knew might see the film and know that they were struggling with their childlessness (or potential childlessness). My friend, as a mother, had never heard women share their stories like this: their shame, isolation, depression, suicidal fantasies, stigma, grief and anger; she had no idea. The fact that these articulate, capable, intelligent women refused to even allow themselves to be filmed, as if they had actually committed a crime, completely blew her mind. She had no idea how shaming it felt to be a childless-by-circumstance woman and although she'd heard me talk about it she didn't really *believe* it until she saw it with her own eyes.

Symbolic Annihilation

From the moment we wake up we are bombarded with images of pregnant women, mothers and children, 'fertile' (ie: young) women, grandmothers and nuclear families. In an article quoting media studies academic Martha M Lauzen, it is reported that:

> ...women in their teens, 20s and 30s are 39 percent of the population, yet are 71 percent of women on TV. Women 40 and older are 47 percent of the population, yet are 26 percent of women on TV.[30]

So, it's not in our imagination that we seem to be invisible. And of those women '40 and older' that *are* on TV, how many of those are childless by either circumstance or choice? And of those, how many of them will be shown as being OK with that and getting on with their childless or childfree lives in happy and meaningful ways? Hmmm, I wonder... Lauzen continues:

> When any group is not featured in the media, they have to wonder, well, what part do I play in this culture? There's actually an academic term for that. It's called 'symbolic annihilation'.[31]

Being a mother (whatever kind of mother you are) gives a woman instant status – it's one of the reasons why socially disadvantaged teenagers become mothers. How many times have you seen a woman interviewed or mentioned in the news as, 'Mother of four, woman X, says...', or 'Woman X, 32, mother of two, said...' By being a mother, these women are automatically given the status of grown-up women with an opinion that matters. I'm not saying that their opinion *doesn't* matter, but it's not the only voice in town. The voice of mothers carries a disproportionate weight compared to that of non-mothers in our culture right now.

After all, how would we understand anything? 'You're not a mother, you wouldn't understand,' is the hurtful unspoken, and sometimes spoken, belief. And indeed, perhaps, in *some* cases we might not. But not *all*.

> We're all human. All experience is valid. And *no one* has a monopoly on understanding.

The gift of empathy (literally 'feeling-into') is what makes it possible for non blood-related humans to live together in society. It makes civilisation possible. We all, to a greater or lesser degree, have the capacity to imaginatively feel what others' lives are like. We don't have to actually *live* those lives to imagine what it might be like for them. After all, this is how art and literature works; we imagine ourselves in another's shoes. It is one of the gifts of humanity and it is not one that childless women are incapable of. Considering that so many of us spent years imagining and dreaming of becoming mothers, we've had plenty of time to imagine how motherhood would be. We've also had information on it shoved in our faces for years, whether we wanted it or not. I think I could write a plausible parenting manual with all the information I've absorbed!

The power of a mother's love for her child has a fierceness that I will never experience first hand. But I have a mother, I was a child once and I've been passionately in love. If I connect the unconditional love I have for my mother with the passionate intensity of romantic love I think I can *imagine* what parental love might feel like. And therefore I can *imagine* how a love of that intensity and permanence might motivate a mother to behave in certain ways.

But how much time, if any, do mothers and others spend wondering what it's like to be us – to be a childless-by-circumstance woman in a motherhood-obsessed culture?

All we ask is that the gift of imaginative empathy be sent our way too. Our experience as childless women is valid and not something to be pushed out of mind as 'distasteful'. For one reason or another, 20% of all women will remain childless, possibly 25% in generations to come, and it's no longer acceptable for us to be treated as freaks of nature.

> Those mothers may have childless daughters one day; they really need to wake up to how they're treating their childless sisters.

Challenging the Stereotypes of Childless Women

As the respect and empathy we crave from mainstream culture may be some time coming, for the time being we can at least change the way *we feel* about ourselves. Just because the culture currently only has a limited set of restrictive and reductive stereotypes for us to fit into, we don't actually have to comply...

This is how all change happens: from the inside out.

When I ask childless women in my groups and workshops to think of as many archetypes, names or roles as they can think of for older, childless women in two minutes, here are the ones they most commonly come up with:

- Spinster, old maid
- Mad old cat lady
- Career woman
- Dried up old bag, bat or hag
- Lesbian

- Childless or maiden aunt

- Witch

- Wicked or evil stepmother

- Etc.

Depressing, isn't it! However, upon closer inspection, I've discovered that if we group these negatives into 'themes', something interesting starts to appear.

It would seem that each one of these negative archetypes, when turned on its head, reveals what this shaming is really all about – the suppression of feminine power.

As the following table shows, each negative and shaming archetype conceals its opposite. But why should feminine power be so threatening that it has to be shamed into silence, into inaction? Perhaps it's because if the power that childless women potentially possess were to be used purposefully and respected culturally it would undermine one of the central planks of patriarchy – namely that men are 'in charge' because they're *inherently more capable of doing so*. When perhaps the reality might be is that the reason men have historically been 'in charge' is because they haven't been bringing up children…

THE HIDDEN POWER WITHIN CHILDLESS WOMEN STEREOTYPES	
STEREOTYPES	**POWER-TYPES**
Spinster or old maid	A woman who has no need of a man to validate her identity
Mad old cat lady	A woman who enjoys her own company and prefers cats to men. (Note: 'Catwoman' in Batman was not called 'Catlady' because 'woman' is a power word, 'lady' is not.)
Career woman	A woman who wields power in the public (male) domain and therefore shows that women are as capable of this as men. (Note: there is no term such as 'career man' not.)
Dried up old bag, bat or hag	A menopausal woman who has moved past allure to a place of deeper wisdom.
Lesbian	A woman who prefers women as sexual and life partners and thus has no need of a male partner.
Childless or maiden aunt	A happy, childless older woman who may act as a role model to a man's children and show that you don't need to be a mother to be fulfilled.
Witch	An older, powerful, knowledgeable woman skilled in life and lore who can fight her own battles. A matriarch, warrior, wise woman and leader.
Wicked or evil stepmother	A woman with influence and power over a man's genetic inheritance.

Reductive archetypes are not *exclusively* used for childless women – we all use them and they act as a useful form of social shorthand. From the 'yummy mummy' to the 'tiger mother', mothers get labelled too, but rarely do their labels contain the spite and shaming power that childless women's archetypes do. Apart from being branded 'a bad mother' perhaps.

In fact, very few of those used to diminish childless women are used to our face, except 'career woman', which proves that those using them *know full well* their power to wound. However, as a tool of ideological control, such negative archetypes have done a good job of making older childless women feel so ashamed of themselves that they've felt uncomfortable embracing the power and freedom that their situation allows.

Although it would take another whole book to fully explore the hidden meanings and suppressed power of the negative archetypes used to shame childless women into submission, for now I wish to explore just a few of them to give us a taste of what's going on underneath the surface.

Spinsters

Whereas 'bachelor' is a term that implies a future, 'spinster' is one loaded with failure. It's as if all possibilities of happiness, of things turning out OK, are quashed by the word 'spinster'.

> Far from being a term of disparagement, originally a spinster was a term of respect and to marry a spinster was to marry a woman who brought an income with her.

This is ironic because the term was first used during the 19th century industrial revolution in Britain to denote a woman who was unmarried and had the profession of 'spinner' – some of the first 'career women' in fact. Spinsters were often the breadwinners for their families as they were able to work from home and combine taking care of other members of the family with earning money.

These days, spinster carries the unstated prefix: 'bitter'. It denotes a woman who is presumed to have been too stupid, unattractive or ambitious to get a partner during her fertile years. Whereas just a generation ago, being an unmarried mother was to be the social outcast, now it's the single, childless woman over 40 who carries the weight of shame. Yet, for some women this is not a situation they chose, but rather one that they've ended up in because they've made intelligent, honourable choices and behaved with decency and morality towards others. Many of them have cared for vulnerable family members through their fertile years, have refrained from getting pregnant 'accidentally' without a partner's consent and have worked hard as members of their families, workplaces and communities and have contributed to society as taxpayers.

When young women today look at how older childless women are ridiculed, what possible message can they take from this except that feminism is bunk? That despite what feminism says, having a family is the *only* guaranteed route to having lasting life-long power and social standing as a woman? And so the status quo and pronatalism score another goal and perhaps lead to yet another woman who might choose to serve her community and her dreams in *other* ways to become a mother without fully thinking it through. And therefore, perhaps, to become a parent who later wishes she hadn't, which isn't great for anyone involved.

Mad Old Cat Lady

More than perhaps any other stereotype, the 'Mad Old Cat Lady' seems to have the power to strike the most fear into the hearts of childless women. So much so that childless women who take pleasure in their pets, as I do (and always have) may try to hide that from people in case they are ridiculed. In the Gateway Women Online Community, I started a section called 'Furbabies' and within hours the Community timeline was a solid wall of fluff. Yet these same women would never have shared these pictures with their friends on Facebook because of the shame they'd feel. 'Oh, so these are baby substitutes?!' people will sneer, unkindly. What's going on here?

Why should childless women with pets (often cats, but plenty of dogs, horses, chickens, etc. too) be made to feel ashamed of this? After all, parents and children have family pets and know how close the bond can be, so why deny this pleasure to childless women?

My feeling is that it may have something to do with the fact that nurturing our pets is extremely rewarding, and that the love and affection that our pets give us in return is not something we 'deserve'. We're meant to be miserable outcasts, not happy pet owners. The way that our pets bond with us in just the same way as they do with other humans perhaps also unconsciously points out that childless women are actually no different from other people! Pets are also a lot less high-maintenance than children and perhaps mothers resent the fact that we don't have the responsibilities of motherhood but are still getting some joy by the back door. I suspect that many mothers feel stitched-up by pronatalism and are finding parenting, for all the social approval they get, much less rewarding and meaningful that they expected. At an unconscious level this may create a resentment towards childless and childfree women which may lead them to subconsciously wish us to be unhappy. Perhaps seeing the uncomplicated and joyful love that passes between our pets and us just doesn't sit well with this. And so they shame us.

I remember a conversation I overheard at a drinks party during the last couple of years of my 'still hopeful' period. A beautiful and talented single childfree-by-choice woman was being pursued by a man who didn't seem to be getting anywhere with her. In frustration he blurted out, 'If you're not careful, you're going to end up as one of those old women living on her own with a load of cats!' And her answer, goddess bless her, was, 'If everything goes to plan.' I laughed out loud and it lodged in my brain as something so unusual I couldn't forget it. It's taken me years to understand how radical it was of her, and how much I admire her for it.

The fact is, there's absolutely nothing to fear about living on your own or having pets. It's not everyone's choice but neither is it such a terrible fate. After all, if you're content on your own and have animals around you to nurture your spirit, what's the big deal? It's power, of course. Because a woman like this is one who has unplugged from the patriarchy – she doesn't need to be someone's wife or mother to be happy, and that's a threat to the status quo. So the very thought of it has been made into a shaming stereotype. Now, I'm not saying that every old woman who lives on her own with cats is happy about that. But neither is every old woman living in her adult children's spare bedroom and having her freedom curtailed by unwanted childcare duties for her grandchildren, blaring music and slamming doors. Both are stereotypes that whitewash the individual reality of each woman's situation. And let's not forget that some of those unhappy old women living on their own with cats might have children who don't bother to visit. It's time to look this stereotype full in the face and refuse to be shamed by it.

Wrapped up in the fear of the 'Mad Old Cat Lady' are other fears – of losing our mind when we're old, of being alone and having no one to care for us and all the fears of old age that lurk at the edges of adult consciousness. Perhaps one of the reasons that this stereotype has such a strong hold is because right now everyone's scared of getting old and what's going to happen. The old way of being old doesn't work anymore and a new way of doing it hasn't yet taken hold. Perhaps by throwing their fear on us, parents feel protected for a moment.

Ageing itself has become a sort of taboo in our culture, no one wants it to happen to them and somehow there's an idea that if we don't talk about it we can avoid it – a collective form of denial. Childless and childfree women are less able than parents to push thoughts of our ageing to one side because we can't kid ourselves that our kids are going to sort this all out later. This is a strength of our position, not a weakness, once we realise that. (More on our fears around ageing without children in Chapter 12.)

If we look this stereotype full in the face and own both its light and shadow aspects, perhaps we can see that all things considered, it might not actually be all that bad a way to live out our twilight years? After all, having learned to live with childlessness, we're probably more equipped to deal with the isolation and issues of old age than many parents. They may have children, but we've got internal resources and a strong social network to support us.

> I live alone, I have a cat. And if I don't have a problem with that, who can use it against me? No one.

Career Woman

Have you ever heard of a man with a job referred to as a 'career man'? No, nor have I.

'Career woman' is a term applied to older childless women who work for a living It's a term that implies that the woman has *chosen* her career over having a family and thus by doing so has proved herself to be 'not all that maternal', which is code for not a 'real' woman. Although, you do have to wonder what other kind of woman there could possibly be apart from 'real' ones!

Now, there are indeed women who recognise that if they want to get to the top of their profession, they're going to have to forgo having children. And if they make that choice, however tinged with regret, it *is* a legitimate choice. Dame Janet Baker, the world-famous British opera singer, said in a 2012 interview in The Guardian: 'I knew, energy wise, I couldn't both bring up children and have a career. And that has never been a decision I have regretted.'[32] However, not all of us have the interest, talent or support to get to the top of our profession, and even childless women doing what they would describe as 'jobs', not 'careers,' are called career women. However, one does have to wonder how many top male opera singers have had to make the same 'choice'…

In March 2012 I was on Irish radio after an interview with me was published in the Irish press.[33] The male presenter referred to me on air as a 'career woman' and I corrected him: 'No,' I said, 'I'm a woman who works. I wanted a family and it didn't work out for me. And in the years that it didn't work out, I carried on working as I needed to earn a living. I did not *choose* work over a family. And now that I've been consistently working, without much interruption, for the last thirty years, it looks like a career.' I could practically hear him rustling his researcher's notes wondering how a sob story about a woman without children had gone all 'feminist'!

> For those of us who are what is now being called 'socially infertile' (not being able to find a suitable partner with whom to have children during our fertile years), to be called a 'career woman' is to imply a degree of choice about the situation that often wasn't there.

The fact is, in order to succeed in the workplace, many more women have become highly educated and often don't even start their professional life until their early to mid-20s. By the time they've learned the skills of their profession and have moved up the ladder, they're 30. At this point, they're still confident of their attractiveness in the marriage market and hope to get married and have children in the next couple of years. But now they face a situation that, as yet, is not really being talked about – 'marrying up'.

The shock absorber generation (as I term it) is living through a transitional time in the relationship between the sexes and carrying some 'old values' (learned from their mothers and the culture) into entirely new situations, where they make an uneasy fit. And 'marrying up' is one of them. In the days when marriage was a woman's only chance to improve her economic status, choosing a partner of a higher social or economic status was a key ambition. Think of Jane Austen novels if you want to recall how crucial it used to be. And the more beautiful or accomplished the young woman, the 'better' she could do for herself.

However, as women went into higher education and the professions in vastly greater numbers, this was *not* matched by a corresponding increase in men doing the same. So now we have a generational situation where many *more* women are looking to choose partners from the same limited pool of high-status men. It is not that there is a drought of 'good men' as some women believe, but that there is a flood of 'good women'.

Add to this that a high-status man will often prefer to partner with a young, attractive woman with plenty of time left on her fertility clock, and we have a situation where many women around the age of 40 are finding themselves still unpartnered or with men who are not 'right' to have a family with.

This 'shock absorber' effect does not work entirely in men's favour though – it only works for high-status men. 'Lower-status men' (what used to be called 'blue-collar' workers) who traditionally would have had no difficulty finding a wife, are similarly being left unpartnered. As many of the women from their own background have become executives and doctors rather than the secretaries and nurses they may have been a generation ago, they are often no longer interested in dating or marrying them.

However, as professional single women move into their mid to late thirties, held fast in the grip of babymania, some of them reluctantly begin to consider these lower-status men as someone they could 'settle for'. The men, perhaps bitter and sore after years of rebuffs and loneliness, are quite likely to reject the women as being 'over the hill' just to get even again. And anyway, who can blame them for not wanting to start a family with someone who's possibly always going to resent them for being 'not quite good enough'? Think of 'Miranda' in the TV series 'Sex and the City' who has a baby with 'Steve', a 'good man' – but so many of their problems as a couple are due to their differing status as professionals vs. blue-collar, college educated vs. street smart.

There are so many interlocking factors that lead to childlessness – unconscious behaviours and out-dated beliefs, mixed with our new way of living and working. We all need to remember that it's only 45 years since we started this experiment after many thousands of years of women being reliant on men economically, and pregnancy being mostly out of women's control. It's going to take a bit of time to work out how to navigate it.

In the meantime, we need to start talking about how these changes are affecting everyone, both men *and* women. We need not take all the blame on our shoulders, nor presume that all men are happy with the unintended consequences of their choices either. Childless women are an easy target because we already bear the shame of the childless taboo, but we don't need to take *all* the blame for the fallout from the biggest shift in relationships between men and women since we moved from the earlier matrilineal to our current patriarchal social structure several thousand years ago.

Aunts

Whilst many of us have nephews, nieces and godchildren, not all of us are as actively involved in their lives as the stereotype of the doting or interfering aunt would suggest. It implies, once again, that we 'lack' something and that we will only fulfil it through a vicarious involvement with other people's children. This in turn reinforces the idea that only children can bring meaning into our lives, which isn't true, although it's such a prevalent one that it's hard to believe that it's just an idea, not a 'truth'.

There is absolutely nothing wrong with being involved in the lives of the children around us – Melanie Notkin, Founder of Savvy Auntie, has coined a great word for it – 'childful'[34] – but it's the act of being *defined* by that involvement that I take issue with.

Being an active aunt, godmother or friend is not a way of compensating for our childlessness; it is an act of love and care for others. To suggest that our love for the young people in our life is some kind of spontaneous compensation mechanism is an insult to all of those women involved in the lives of children not their own. And an insult to the children and young people as well. Ours is a loving and voluntary choice, not purely a way to fulfil a biological need.

Wrapped up in the 'doting aunt' stereotype of the fussy older childless woman clucking around children, doling out sweeties and patting them on the head, is a kind of chocolate-box patronisation. The stereotypical childless aunt is not some va-va-voom exciting, glamorous grown-up, but rather a sexless, shapeless and harmless free babysitter. This stereotype devalues both the real contribution so many childless women (blood-related or not) make to the lives of children and the nature of the relationship. We are not free babysitters and cake-makers – we are that 'village of elders' that children need as they grow to maturity. We offer a different take on life from their mothers and peers, one that they seek and value us for.

Only very recently my 16 year-old niece asked me, 'If nobody likes feminists why are *you* one?' This started a fascinating conversation which continued on Facebook as I directed her towards various age-appropriate resources that I felt might help to counter the cultural rubbishing of women's power she's been exposed to. I don't think she'd ever have asked her mother the same question.

LESBIANS

In a 2012 article by comedian Chloe Hilliard titled: 'I'm Not a Lesbian, I'm Just Childless', Hilliard writes:

> *I'm 31 years old, black and childless. Coming from an American-American family with strong southern roots, that means either I can't have kids or I'm a lesbian.*[35]

Newsflash! First and foremost, lesbians are actually *women*. Whoa – hold onto your hats folks! They have the same fertility window as heterosexual women, the same infertility issues and, for those of them who hope to be mothers, the same issues in finding the 'right' relationship to bring a family into. Some of them also are with partners who already have children from earlier relationships and so many of them face the 'childless-by-relationship' issue too.

Sometimes, calling a childless woman a lesbian is a way of insulting her, of suggesting that she's either too 'strident' (i.e. has a mind of her own) or too 'ugly' to 'get a man', because that's what conservative culture still thinks of lesbians – that they're not 'real women'. Whilst the LGBT community has been steadily becoming more visible for years now, the journey for childless/childfree women has only just begun. We have a lot to learn from them, in particular how they have reclaimed many of the words that used to be insults, as well as supporting each other and forming a tribe. And being prepared to call out prejudice and refusing to be shamed into silence by the insults thrown at them.

> Being a single childless woman doesn't mean you're a lesbian, it's wanting to spend the rest of your life with a woman you love passionately that does.

Unlike heterosexual women, people don't automatically jump to the conclusion that lesbian women already have children or *must* want to have children soon. The hidden prejudice here is that by *not* being heterosexual, lesbian women aren't 'real' women (aren't you getting tired of all the ways we can somehow not be 'real' women!) and that therefore they're obviously not going to be maternal.

Whilst perhaps it might possibly be a relief *not* to get bombarded with the 'When are you going to have a baby?' or, 'How many kids have you got?' questions, in other ways, it's a double-negative discounting of lesbians as women. Not thinking of them as possible mothers is yet another way of 'othering' them from mainstream society.

WICKED STEPMOTHERS

Did a chill just run through you at the words 'wicked stepmother'? The image of the childless woman as threatening to a child's very existence is one of the most potent of all the shaming stereotypes that can be projected onto childless women as it includes a double dose of shame: bad mother *and* childless woman. This 'wickedness' is projected most strongly onto childfree women, who are often considered to be unnatural (not 'real women' again!) in their active choice not to have children. Childless-by-circumstance women are often presumed to have chosen this outcome and so we too get tarred with the same ridiculous brush. However, even if others *know* that we are childless-by-circumstance, the taboo nature of our situation carries *such* weight that we too may subconsciously be considered unnatural and therefore, in some subtle way, touched by evil, by wickedness.

As more than one childless woman has told me, people have suggested to them that obviously they were not 'fit' to be mothers in some way and that God knew that! And some of those comments have come from members of the clergy or other organised religions.

To be a stepmother is, in some sense, to accept that you are the wrong woman in the wrong place at the wrong time for your partner's children. When you are also childless yourself (not always by choice – sometimes your partner doesn't want more children or it's just not possible for a whole host of reasons) being a stepmother is doubly hard. If you get very close to your step-children you'll be accused of trying to usurp their mother's role and if the relationship with them is stormy, it'll be because you're not a mother yourself *so you obviously don't know what the hell you're doing.* The fact that the relationship with your partner's children is difficult because the kids themselves have been placed in a difficult position doesn't often seem to be acknowledged. There are various online forums for childless stepmothers (see Appendix) and over and over again I can see how women feel that they are made to feel that they don't have a voice in the family situation, even though they are doing a huge amount of the parenting. Sue Fagalde Lick's book 'Childless by Marriage'[36] writes movingly and candidly of marrying a man who decided after they married that he'd already completed his family. She and her husband loved each other dearly, but being a stepmother looks like it can be the world's most thankless task as a childless woman.

In fairy tales, the Evil or Wicked Stepmother is a kind of witch who, by her very existence, seems to have stolen the children's rightful mother and be in competition for their father's love. So therefore she's going to want to get rid of them as soon as possible. In order to be truly evil (think Snow White's stepmother) she also needs to be childless, so that she's one of those unnatural women to whom nature 'wisely' gave no children. If she was a mother herself, it would be harder to make her truly evil, as it would fight against the stereotype of mothers as good and selfless.

Witches

The fear of the childless woman has deep roots in our culture. If you think of both modern and ancient fairy tales, whether it's the evil scheming of Snow White's stepmother Queen or the self-obsession, vanity and insanity of Cruella de Vil in 101 Dalmatians, older childless women are *never* the heroines. Things rarely end well for them!

This cultural prejudice against older childless women goes back to a time when women's knowledge as healers, herbalists and midwives became feared by the church, as it was the continuation of ancient pagan knowledge from pre-Christian times. In a time when having a large family was the only way to ensure that you had enough labour for your land and that you would be taken care of in old age, when childbirth was perilous and infant mortality high, local healers had enormous prestige. They were also slightly feared, as they were 'apart' (different) from other women.

Often living without a family and on the edge of villages (apart from others) they were consulted by local leaders for their wisdom. It is thought that such healers and midwives had knowledge of herbs to prevent pregnancies and ease deliveries, as well as to promote fertility or cause a miscarriage. The power invested in these 'wise women' was revered and feared by men and their knowledge was passed on orally. In a time before literacy, experienced older people were the libraries of their time, and valued and revered for this.

During the Renaissance in Europe, such knowledge began to be seen as in direct competition with the rise of science and the rule of the organised church. Wise women and midwives were branded as 'witches' and hunted down and killed. It is estimated that 200,000 witches were accused and 100,000 were executed – either burnt alive or drowned – during the witch hunts of the 17th century, although accurate records are difficult to find.[37] It was a female holocaust, eradicating both ancient knowledge and putting a fear of feminine power and mystery at the very centre of modern patriarchy and culture.

> From the eradication of powerful women (and goddesses) from the Bible, including the writings that showed that the Hebrew God Yahweh had a wife and consort called Asherah[38] through to the destruction of pagan fertility goddesses by the spread of Christianity and the burning of witches, feminine power and mystery have been shamed into silence and erased from history.

Only youth and motherhood have retained any prestige as they serve to protect male interests. We have lived for so long under patriarchy (literally 'the rule of the father') that it seems normal to live like this, but it's a worn-out system.

A much more egalitarian way of viewing both men and women is needed today. A system which shames, sidelines and ignores 1:5 women from their 40s onwards and therefore keeps them at the margin of society, unable to contribute in productive ways, is not just unfair, it's unsustainable and counter-productive to the development of our culture.

However, change takes time, and courage. There is an expression, 'courage in a woman is often mistaken for insanity', which says it all really! We can stay quiet and out of sight (and miserable) or make a noise and risk being thought nuts. Having tried the former and almost disappeared with sadness, I now choose the latter.

Choose Your Own Label

Once you start using the Internet to connect with other women without children, you discover that there are a lot of terms and labels to describe us. Childless, childfree, CBC (childless-by-choice), CNBC (childless-not-by-choice) DINKS (double-income-no-kids), PANKS (professional-aunt-no-kids), GINKS (green inclinations no kids), Unparents, childful, notmoms, barren, sterile, infertile…

I came up with the term NoMo (not-mother) because I wanted one that didn't include the word 'child', could be applied to *any* woman without children and sounded a bit groovy, like the latest hip part of New York. It's an abbreviation of 'not-mother', or 'non-mother', as you like. It can be used for both childless and childfree women but, like all terms, it will find its own way in the world and may stick or not. At first, I didn't think about it being used for *all* women without children, but journalists have picked up on it that way and that's how it's been used in the media.[39] Time will tell.

Some of us hate the term 'NoMo' and prefer 'Gateway Woman' (which I like, of course). And many childless women disagree strongly with the notion of having a label at all.

In my blog 'The Gateway Women Manifesto: Are Childless Women the New Suffragettes?' I wrote:

> *Yes, I know it's annoying that we need a 'label' at all…*
> *Interestingly, the suffragettes thought so too – the term*
> *was coined by that famously 'women-friendly' newspaper*
> *the Daily Mail to ridicule members of the Women's*
> *Social and Political Union. Which they then reclaimed*
> *and made their own. No one uses the term suffragette*
> *anymore. Why? Because their work is done and we accept*
> *that women have as much right to vote as men. So we*
> *don't need the 'label' anymore*[40]

As childless women, we are outsiders in the culture. I understand the women who don't want a label apart from 'woman'. But sometimes we need to give up a little bit of our individuality to create some solidarity – to show how many we are and what we're really like.

If you don't want a label, fine. But consider this: perhaps by *not* finding one that you feel OK about identifying with, you're actually participating in the silent shaming that perpetuates our outsider status? We've got nothing to be ashamed of. The fact is, others have given you a label and they use it when you're not listening – wouldn't you rather choose your own?

To name something is a powerful thing. It creates a reality. It owns it. Just as homosexual men and women have reclaimed 'gay', 'queer' and 'dyke' as terms that *they* define the meaning for, not others, childless-by-circumstance women who won't be silenced or shamed by how things have turned out for them now need a term to rally behind. When we find one that the vast majority of us feel comfortable with and proud of, we'll already be halfway to not needing it anymore.

Exercise 5: Role Models

Collect any images you can find in the media of childless women, particularly women 45+ for whom childlessness is most likely to be permanent. Sort the images into categories / stereotypes.

Here are a few questions for you to ponder:

- What sort of ratio can you find between positive and negative stereotypes?

- Are most of the women childfree or childless – or is it difficult to know their story?

- Is there a derogatory name, label or archetype for older childless women that you fear being applied to you?

- Of the stereotypes you've identified, can you identify the 'light' aspect of it (ie: the hidden power) underneath the negative, insulting, 'shadow' side?

- Is there an older, childless or childfree woman you admire in your family, community, workplace or in the public eye? What is it about her that speaks to you? Can you think of a way to open a dialogue with her?

- How do you feel about childfree-by-choice women? Is there anything you think about them that you wouldn't want people to think about you? Are you perhaps prejudiced towards them in ways that you fear people are prejudiced against you? Can you see that it might not be true?

- What label do you choose for yourself? Even if you don't want one you've already got one; it's just that others probably don't use it to your face. It might be 'that sad woman who couldn't have kids and never got over it', or 'that witch from accounts'. Wouldn't you rather people started using a label you've chosen for yourself?

Reflections on this Chapter

In this chapter we've explored how childless women are perceived in the culture and, in turn, how we perceive ourselves. Sometimes, beginning to lift the lid on this stuff can be quite explosive, so if you've found yourself getting a bit hot under the collar over the last week, that's quite normal...

If you did the 'Role Models' exercise, you may have found yourself astonished by how narrow and negative the view is that the media (which is the amplifier of the culture) has of childless women.

You may begin to notice the language that other people use and you may see changes in the language that you use yourself. Also, you may being to reflect on how other stigmatised or marginalised groups might feel about the way that they are spoken to, or about...

As we begin to realise how the ways in which we are viewed (and have viewed ourselves) may have contributed to our own unhappiness, we may be quite shocked and even feel quite foolish. It's important not to shame ourselves for this – we've done quite enough of that already.

Now you are beginning to see the world around you more clearly you can make some different choices, which will bring with them sometimes unwelcome, but ultimately liberating, responsibilities. As Eleanor Roosevelt is famously quoted as saying: 'No one can insult you without your permission.' A big part of getting your mojo back as a childless woman is to reclaim your power and identity as a woman who matters. If others don't agree, that's not our problem anymore!

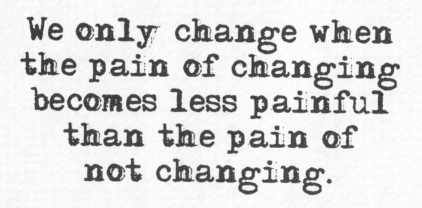

We only change when
the pain of changing
becomes less painful
than the pain of
not changing.

CHAPTER 6

WHO MOVED MY MOJO?

DUSTING OFF YOUR DANCING SHOES

After all the years of hoping, presuming, trying, crying, grieving, raging and coping with the whole damn 'baby thing', you probably wouldn't recognise your mojo if it came up to you and asked you to dance! And even then, you'd probably refuse. Dance? You must be out of your mind... I don't do *that* any more!

You may wonder if, after all you've been through, you actually *want* to find your mojo again. Sounds exhausting just thinking about it, doesn't it, let alone actually doing something about it... You feel sluggish, worn-out and done-in. You stay busy, *too busy*, at work but at home you can't be bothered to do much at all. You're behind with all your life admin and surrounded by half painted walls, unfinished projects and piles of books you can't quite get around to reading. You don't really have a social life anymore, which is quite a relief as you'd be embarrassed for anyone to see how you really live these days...

It doesn't feel like a promising place from which to start anything, does it?

After all, isn't this whole mojo thing a bit fanciful? Another bit of new age mumbo-jumbo to get your hopes up, only to leave you one book heavier and back where you started? Why bother?

> Well, you always have the option to stay exactly where you are.

And in fact you may *need* to stay there until you *can't* stay there any more. In my own experience, change isn't something any of us undertakes because it seems like a good idea. Well, not change that sticks anyway. Because it seems that we only change when the pain of *not* changing becomes more painful than the pain of changing.

Being wary of change is part of human nature. I watched a TED video of a Tony Robbins talk[41] in which he asks the audience if they like surprises: 'Yes!' they chorus (this is a TED audience after all). 'Bullshit!' he replies, 'You like the surprises you enjoy, the rest you call problems!' That sounds about right to me.

Change is not something we find easy because change is something our ego sees as a risk factor and being risk-averse is a good biological survival strategy. However, we need our ego, no matter how much of a rough ride it gets in a lot of self-help literature; without it we'd be unable to function in the world and would have to be locked up for our own and others' safety. Our ego is a filtering and organising system that works out which parts of the endless stream of data coming our way are relevant and which aren't. What's a threat and what's not. Who we are, and who we aren't. Its function is to make sense out of nonsense – to sift and filter all the incoming data from our senses and create a comprehensible version of reality that keeps us safe and meets our needs. As far as the ego is concerned, any non-essential randomness (ie: change) is to be avoided as it increases risk.

The ego is also the part of our consciousness that creates our identity and gives us a sense of who we are compared to other people. It's always in flux, always assessing new data and accepting or rejecting the information as it fits with our prevailing idea *at the time* of who we are and what's important to us. Do you remember how it was when you longed to be pregnant and all you could see were pregnant women everywhere? That was your ego highlighting what was important to you at the time. It wasn't that fate had decided to put more pregnant women in your path just to break your heart a little bit more, even though it may have felt like it at the time.

Although it's beyond the scope of this book to explore the nature of the ego in depth, it's relevant here because realising that the idea of having a fixed identity, a 'me' who never changes, is actually an *illusion* can help to allay some of our fears that transitioning into a new Plan B identity isn't possible. You've already had many different 'identities' in your life so far. If you think about it, isn't your sense of 'yourself' today different from what it was when you were a child or a young woman? And yet, at the time, wouldn't you have said that these identities were absolutely 'you'? That's how the ego works; it presents a snapshot in time as something unchanging, but it's not true. It's an illusion, a mind-trick, a technique our consciousness has evolved to help us cope with the ever-changing nature of reality.

One of the reasons that losing something or someone we consider vital to our sense of self is so painful is that the ego experiences it as an attack on our own identity, on our sense of who we think we are. I hope this helps to understand why losing the potential identity of 'mother' can be so very hard to cope with. As so many of us know, you don't have to actually *be* a mother in order to have a huge part of our identity invested into the goal or role of motherhood.

> The grieving process is one where, like love, our identity shifts. We are never the same person again after loving someone or losing someone.

When we fall in love, our brain is flooded with chemicals that pretty much keep the ego too drunk to notice the radical structural renovations it's undertaking. With grief, denial is the mechanism that keeps the show on the road until your ego is ready to begin the shift to this new identity.

However, during the process of grieving (which is an active process, rather than the passive 'stuckness' of grief) there is a fluidity to our sense of self which offers us the chance to reconsider whether being fixated on our identity serves us in the long run. It's a transformational time, an opportunity to build a relationship with the 'witnessing' part of us that runs much deeper than our ego – the core part of our consciousness from which our ego developed. This is what meditation practices are for, but you don't need to meditate to take this first step – just wondering who it is who is able to think about things like 'identity' and 'ego'. Who is this witness? Learning to notice this calm and more spacious part of ourselves can be the beginning of developing a more flexible approach to life. This can make the twists and turns of fate much easier to bear.

These days, I imagine myself as a tree with well-nourished roots. When storms come, as they always do, these days I bend with the wind. I don't resist the wind anymore, pretend it's not there, yell at it, get depressed by it or feel outraged because I don't deserve it. It's just wind and I just bend. Sometimes, if I'm feeling a bit brittle and resistant *Not fair! Not now! Not my turn! Not mine!* I might snap a few branches, but more and more often I just bend as the storm passes through me. There was a time when I used to joke that the universe had put a sign on my back that read 'kick me'. These days, I don't take life personally. It just is what it is. Except on the days when I don't – I'm not special or different from anyone else, I'm like you, like all of us, a work in progress. And there are days when my ego runs the show, and it's not pretty.

Your ego, your psyche, will change when it has to, when you're ready, and not a moment sooner. It might be that by reading this book you are laying the ground for change at a later date, or it might be that something in this book provides the catalyst you need to start changing. You may have already started.

Trust yourself. Yes *you*, really. If you're not ready to make any changes yet, don't give yourself a hard time about it. It's not going to help and it won't speed things up. Your timing is just that; your timing. You can feed and water a plant and place it in the sun, but you can't make it grow any quicker than it grows.

Wisdom is precious because of the price we pay for it.

So we're going to start with some remembering; a gentle process of remembering who you were before motherhood seemed to become something that was slipping out of your grasp. Yes, there was a time when you had other dreams, other ambitions apart from being a mother – whether you came to this idea late or whether you spent decades writing names in baby books.

Now, I'm not saying that you need to go backwards; but rather that within those old dreams, those half-remembered memories are clues that will lead you, in your own time, towards your own Plan B.

CREATING A LIFE OF MEANING

In 1946, Viktor Frankl, a Viennese psychiatrist interned by the Nazis in various concentration camps, wrote a short memoir describing his experiences and outlining what was to become 'logotherapy' – a form of existential psychotherapy which focuses on finding a reason to live. At the time of his death in 1997, 'Man's Search for Meaning' had been translated into 24 languages and had sold over 10 million copies.[42]

This short book, which can be read in an afternoon, is life-changing. It's a book about the power of the human spirit to survive, and even flourish, when every conceivable human right, need and dignity has been taken away. It's about the choice we all have, as human beings, in *any* situation, to decide how we are going to feel about it. To decide what meaning we are going to give it. In the book, Frankl quotes the philosopher Nietzsche in that, 'He who has a why to live can endure almost any how.' Make that a 'she'.

Because without a 'why', even the most luxurious and comfortable existence can be a daily torment. You can count your blessings till the cows come home but without a reason, a purpose for living, living itself can become a chore.

I know that you know what I mean. A chore.

It is perhaps only other childless-by-circumstance women who can understand the depth of existential despair that many of us experience, and which leaves us wondering if we have the courage to face the rest of our lives feeling like this. It is a dark night of the soul of such profundity that, if faced and transcended, creates a depth of psychological maturity and compassion in us that very few other adults around us can match. We have looked our death-in-life in the face and survived it. We live with the ashes of invisible dreams, haunted by ghosts that no one but us ever knew.

Finding a way to create a life of meaning from this is an act of great moral courage and absolutely essential if we are to enjoy, rather than merely endure, the rest of our life.

Frankl's book, and the school of existential psychotherapy that he founded, shows that finding the meaning of life is a unique journey for each of us. No one has the answer for you, no one can tell you what your meaning is. And most of us don't even know what it is until we find it. Finding your meaning is like falling in love; you know it when it happens.

As well as being a gift to ourselves, finding and creating a life of meaning is a gift to those around us and to the wider world. Hopefully we've all met people whose lives are shaped in a way that allows them to express what's most important to them. They shine in a way that others don't, and they give courage and hope to all they meet. We live in cynical times, but when we meet someone who has learned how to make their soul sing, ours sings too.

We have a choice.

When we are ready, we can create our new life around something that makes us feel alive in the way that we were convinced *only* having a child could. Or we can flounder for years, never really living, just existing. We can ossify around the identity of 'that woman who didn't have kids and never really got over it' or we can fashion a new one.

You'll know when you're ready to make this transition and there's no shame in taking your time. It takes as long as it takes and shortcuts don't work – I have the mileage on the clock to prove it! Grieving is an exhausting process and change requires energy. You may need some more time to top up your reserves.

Far from planning this, if your experience is anything like mine, you'll realise in retrospect that you've already taken the first step. This is not something you can put on a 'to do' list or schedule – just as you cannot schedule falling in love. But what you *can* do is your groundwork, so that when that moment comes, you're ready. And that's what this book is for.

WHATEVER HAPPENED TO DESPERATELY SEEKING SUSAN?

If I cast my mind back to what I was like in my early twenties, I think I was probably rather scary. Very tall, striking looking and with a bravado mask of bullish confidence that hid my utter cluelessness about who I was. An adult in physical form only. My role model was the character Madonna played in *Desperately Seeking Susan*, a film which came out in 1985 when I was turning 21. I went to the cinema over and over again to see the film, so stunned was I by this radically new idea of how to 'be' a woman. Susan/Madonna was totally unlike anything else I'd seen up until that point in my life. She was ballsy, independent, fearless and sexy and seemed to be running her life just the way *she* wanted it.

After a childhood where I'd learned was that your happiness as a woman was largely dictated by the behaviour of the men in your life, Susan/Madonna's complete disregard for men's opinions, her offhand treatment of their affection and her disregard for the rules of society intoxicated me. Now, although I couldn't sing and had no desire to be a pop-star, I was thrilled and inspired by Susan/Madonna as she busted her way out of what women were 'allowed' to do, think or say and, encouraged and inspired by that, I took life head on, artfully-ripped fishnet tights and all!

Fast-forward around 20 years to my late 30s and I'd been through the tumble-dryer of life: I'd seen bad things happen to good people; saw the love of my life succumb to a heartbreaking drink and drug addiction; suffered a major work-related industrial injury in my late 20s that threw my career trajectory completely out of the window; spent my 30s suffering from unexplained infertility and watching our business, home and marriage be consumed by my husband's addictions (and my co-dependency). I ended up on the floor, literally and metaphorically, a nervous wreck at 38.

Picking myself up from that, fuelled by babymania and with total confidence (ie: in complete denial) that at the age of 40, and after 11 years of 'unexplained infertility' that I'd be remarried and a mother (via IVF) in a couple of years, I propelled myself into new world of online dating. And with babymania as the fuel in my rocket-propelled dating engine, I made some very bizarre decisions with regard to my career, finances and relationships over the next few years.

Coming out of the tunnel of denial at 43½ (the only people other than children under ten who count their years in halves are women running out of time to conceive) *I had no idea who I was anymore.* If someone had said to me at that point that what I needed to do was to construct a new identity around a life of meaning, I think I would have looked at them, understood the words, but not have had a clue what they were talking about.

But one thing I absolutely knew for sure was that what had excited me in my 20s wasn't going to do it for me anymore – for goodness sake, even Madonna had married an Englishman and taken up hunting! However, I seriously doubted if I had the energy to get excited about anything ever again, frankly: I'd try reading books and lose interest after about 50 pages; I'd go to art galleries or museums and all I could think about was getting to the coffee bar and having some cake. I felt about a thousand years old and bored of life. Bored of myself and dangerously uninspired.

Dreams? Goals? Ambitions? Practically none left. I was a spent force, an empty vessel. An ageing and defective woman, alone in her 40s, broke physically, financially, emotionally and spiritually.

However, gradually I began to realise that what had happened is not that I didn't have any dreams anymore, but that I'd *neglected* them for so long that I'd forgotten *how* to have them.

> It also took a great deal of courage to start imagining a future again because deep down I was terrified of dreaming again; the dream of marriage and family had cost me so dear, it seemed too risky to dare to dream of *anything*, ever again.

I genuinely thought that another disappointment, another failure, would finish me off completely so it seemed safer not to even try.

I felt stuck, with no idea how to move forwards. And so I started where I always start, with my first love, writing. For a couple of years, I just journalled but I was *bored* with the sound of my voice on paper, *bored to tears* of the inside of my head. So then I tried blogging and it seemed that the notion that I was potentially writing for someone other than myself, even just *one* reader, helped me to reconnect with my inner storyteller – the mystical, philosophical and cheeky little girl I'd once been and who I felt I'd lost. But she was still in there, waiting for me.

I discovered that even though I felt ancient and almost suffocated by grief-related depression, my capacity to dream had not been completely extinguished. It may have been a whisper of a flame but my pilot light was still on.

And so is yours. Because you wouldn't still be reading if it weren't...

EXERCISE 6: RUSSIAN DOLLS

Grab a pile of Post-It notes. Write each word or phrase that comes to mind in response to this exercise on a separate Post-It note (or separate small pieces of paper).

Imagine yourself as if you were a series of Russian dolls, with the biggest doll being the 'you' you are today, and the smallest doll being the 'you' you were when you were born. Each and every 'you' lives on as a part of you today, along with her hopes and dreams.

Although right now it may feel that the hopeful dreamer in you is well and truly vanquished, I'd like to suggest that she's still in there somewhere. In fact, there's proof: take a moment to recall what it's like when you smell something that instantaneously transports you back to a childhood memory – in that moment, you *are* that age again, with all its rich, vivid aliveness.

Here are three questions to help you connect with three of your Russian dolls – you at three different stages of your girlhood:

- Around the age of five (or just starting your first school)

- Around the age of ten (or just before puberty)

- Around the age of fifteen (or just becoming a young woman)

Write the answers to each of the following questions separately. The prompts below don't necessarily *all* have to be answered – they're just ways to remind you of the kinds of things you may (or may not) have been doing at each age.

Question 1: *What did you love doing when you were a young girl?*

Position: Get onto the floor to answer these – cross-legged or any position that's comfortable. Try to 'see' the world from the height you were when you were around the age of five or six.

1. What did you want to 'be' or 'do' when you grew up?
2. Did you play 'mother and baby' or did you think dolls were silly?
3. Did you like to play alone in nature or stay indoors with friends?
4. Did you like building things with Lego and if so, what did you build?
5. Did you like painting and drawing and if so, what did you paint or draw?
6. Were you an avid reader and storyteller?
7. Were you physically very competent – riding a bike and climbing trees younger than most, or more timid and needing encouragement to try new things?
8. Did you take every chance to be in the kitchen with your mother (or another adult) learning to cook?
9. Were you a tomboy or a princess?
10. Did you lie on your back and gaze at the clouds and think about the nature of reality?
11. Did you grow things in your garden?
12. Did you love dressing up in your mother's clothes and putting on makeup?

Question 2: What did you love doing just before puberty?

Position: Lie on your stomach, sit in a swing, curl up in an armchair – whatever position you can remember being your 'thinking' position when you were around 10 or 11 (or before your periods started).

1. Did you like making things with your hands? If so, what kind of things?

2. Did you like 'homemaking' hobbies like quilting, sewing, cooking, etc?

3. Were you in the Girl Guides or Girl Scouts and if so, what aspect of it did you like?

4. Did you run wild in nature with your friends?

5. Were you a daredevil or a more bookish girl?

6. Did you enjoy being around babies and children and being 'maternal' towards them?

7. Did you read teenage magazines and want to be grown up?

8. Did you think about your future family and have someone you talked about as being the person you were going to marry and have children with one day?

9. Did you read fantasy stories and if so, what did you dream of being – a witch, a princess, a talking horse, an angel, an amazon, a mermaid, an adventurer, an avenger?…

10. Were you in a gang? What was your role?

11. What was your 'role' in your family by this time? The difficult one, the bookish one, the caring one, the problem one, the goody-goody one, etc.

12. Did you have something you wanted to 'do' or 'be' when you grew up?

Question 3: *What did you enjoy (or not) about school?*

Position: Sit at a desk in a hard chair. Try to sit in the position that feels like the one you would have sat in at school when you were around the age of fifteen.

1. Was there a subject that you loved but weren't very good at so you dropped it?

2. Was there a subject that you took extra care with when you did your homework?

3. Was there a teacher that you remember as particularly inspiring? What subject did they teach?

4. Did you hate lessons, but love a different aspect of school? Sport, socialising, music, debating, chess, amateur dramatics, gossip?

5. Was there an out-of-school activity you were more inspired by? A book club, sports club, Girl Guides, etc?

6. What 'crowd' did you hang around with, or were you a loner?

7. If you were a loner, what was different about you, and were you OK with that?

8. Were you a natural leader, a bit of a rebel or perhaps the peacemaker?

9. Did you wish there were subjects you could study that weren't available at your school, or that 'girls' didn't do?

10. If you hated school and bunked off a lot, do you know what it was about school you hated? What did you do when you weren't in school?

11. Did you long for the holidays or were you counting the days till the return to school?

12. If you could have your schooldays over again, what would you do differently?

Take a look at the answers to all three questions at the same time. If they're on Post-It notes or pieces of paper, see if you can start putting answers or ideas together that seem to have similarities.

- Can you see any themes emerging?

- How do you feel when you think about those themes?

- Can you feel a tickle of joy in your gut when you think about one or some of them?

- Notice if you feel fear or any other strong emotion about any of them – this may be a clue that you are attracted to it, but that you may have learnt to be nervous of excitement or joy.

BABY STEPS

Anything that gives you a tingle of joy or even remembered joy is important to pay attention to. Human beings are meaning-making machines, and one of the clues that leads us towards our meaning is joy. When we were children we naturally gravitated towards those things that brought us joy – we found them meaningful, even if no one else agreed with us. As adults many of us have lost that simple connection to meaning; buried it under 'shoulds' and 'musts' until we find it hard to know what moves us anymore. We also make judgements and criticisms of ourselves such as, 'It's ridiculous for a grown woman to enjoy_____' (insert whatever thing you just thought of!)

When I was a young girl, I used to look at grown-ups and think, *They've got as much pocket money as they want, they can go to bed when they want, they can read what they want, they can eat what they want... so why are they all so miserable?* It's amusing, but it's also something that we forget as adults – we're much more in charge of our happiness that we realise...

The grief of childlessness can rob us of our capacity to take joy in the things we used to like. We can be stuck in unprocessed grief for so long that it begins to feel like a permanent character change. Add to this the hormonal changes of peri-menopause, and you can end up in a joyless funk that lasts for years.

Whilst you can't *force* yourself to see life's pleasures again if you're still processing your grief, what you can do is to *start* doing the work to uncover your joy. As we learned earlier, grief is a spiral – not a series of linear steps – and it may be that you can cope with a small dose of joy now, and work up to a life full of joy as the loving energy of grief heals you and prepares you to open up to the world again.

Sometimes, we have to meet life halfway. Show that we're willing to change and then allow ourselves to be changed. You just have to take that first baby step.

> Forget your to-do lists and all the 'grown up' things you need to get done before you can even *consider* doing something 'just for fun'. On the day you die, there will still be things left to do on your to-do list.

But by gently opening your heart to joy again now, you stand a chance of dying as a woman who lived a life that fed her soul, rather than someone who put off her joy in order to get her chores done.

Exercise 7: Baby Steps towards Meaning

Take a look at some of the ideas that the Russian Doll exercise brought up for you – some of the things that you felt that tickle of joy (or fear) about. Is there a way that you could bring a little bit of this into your life over the next week? Nothing huge, but something that takes you towards joy or deep satisfaction.

It might be as small as baking a cake or as big as enquiring about going back to study a subject you once loved. It can be getting back in touch with an old friend or getting your bike out of the garage. It might be buying a new sketch book and doing a drawing for yourself or switching off the TV and going for a swim instead.

Make it as small and as easy to do as possible and commit to it.

Expect some (or a lot!) of resistance to following this through. If you don't manage to do it in the next week, write down all the reasons you came up with as to why you couldn't do it and don't feel ashamed. This is a big challenge to your ego and it may not let you get away with it first time. It's not failure, it's feedback.

REFLECTIONS ON THIS CHAPTER

In this chapter we've started to explore the reasons behind why creating a life of meaning for ourselves as childless women isn't some kind of self-indulgent way to fill the time but is actually a way to save our lives.

How did the ideas about change and resistance work for you? Did you start to realise that it might be possible for you to let go of your identity as an unhappily childless woman? Or did you find that rather challenging? Or perhaps a bit of both!

What came up for you when you did the 'Russian Dolls' exercise? How was it to revisit all those younger versions of yourself? In my experience, when we excavate our past like this, it can bring up a mixture of hope and sadness. Sadness is part of adjusting to loss and deserves to be acknowledged too.

If you did the 'Baby Steps Towards Meaning' exercise – well done! How did it feel to open that tiny little window in your soul and let some fresh air in? Did it give you just the teensiest bit of hope that perhaps, in time, you might be able to be happy again? Or did that taste of happiness scare you, by reminding you how very far you've gone from your true self? And did it perhaps make you sad to realise how hard it is, right now, to give yourself a treat and do something that you enjoy…

All of these feelings, and others, are quite normal. It's usually the meaning, the 'story' we attach to our feelings that causes the problem. Imagine for a moment that you'd been sitting in a darkened room for some time, longing for daylight. When it came, that longed-for sun on your face would be too bright, perhaps even painful. But it wouldn't mean that you'd want to go back into the dark again. You'd squint, and wait for your eyes to adjust… It's the same for us as we move towards our Plan B.

If you tried to do the 'Baby Step Towards Meaning', but found that despite your best intentions, you found a whole host of reasons not to follow through with it – also well done! Not doing the activity gives you a lot of precise feedback to enable you to recalibrate and try again. It might be that you made your Baby Step too worthy, too sensible or too ambitious – and thus it was hard to find the impetus to do it. Have another go – there's no rush. And don't bother giving yourself a hard time for not doing it. It won't get you there any faster. In fact, it'll slow you down and shut you down.

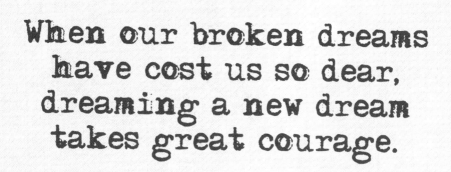

When our broken dreams
have cost us so dear,
dreaming a new dream
takes great courage.

CHAPTER 7

LETTING GO OF YOUR BURNT OUT DREAMS

THE SHADOW OF THE LIFE UNLIVED

When I knew for sure that I was never going to have a biological child of my own I became acutely aware that for many years I'd been living two lives: one in which I was hoping for a baby and making the best of things till then, the other in which I had succeeded and had become a mother.

I call the life I wasn't living, my 'shadow life'. I was, in fact, a 'shadow mother'.

At no point in that time (a 15-year stretch no less) did I fully and completely embrace the life I was *actually* living – that of a childless woman. I was always in transition to the next stage when my *real* life would begin. As a result my reality often felt like a poor fit, but I ascribed my unhappiness and dissatisfaction to the fact that I *wasn't a mother*, rather than it being the very *wanting to be a mother* that was making me miserable. In Buddhism, it is said that the root of all human suffering is 'craving'. Recovering from the pain of childlessness I came to understand that the root of my unhappiness wasn't that I didn't give birth to my longed-for child, but the *craving* I'd had for that child.

I don't doubt that I wanted a child and that I would have been delighted to have become a mother. However, I was totally unable to entertain the idea that I could be happy if that *didn't* work out. Even thinking about it felt disloyal, as if it would make it less likely to happen.

Like so many of us I became so obsessed with having a child, over such a long period of time, that I stopped examining *why* I wanted this, or even whether it was *really true* anymore. It feels terrible to write that, even now. It feels disloyal to myself, my dreams and the family I longed for. And it's precisely that irrational fear (ie: denial) that prevented me from re-examining my dreams and options when I started dating again after my divorce. I was so *familiar* with being obsessed with becoming a mother that I went head-first into looking for a new life partner who was willing to do IVF with me (and had the funds to do so) before time ran out. I reassessed everything *else* about my life but I left my dream of becoming a mother untouched and unexamined.

Gripped by babymania, I made some truly awful decisions about relationships, careers and finances – the aftermath of which I'm still dealing with. By being too afraid to hold my dream of motherhood up to the light in case I lost it, I kept myself in the dark about who I was and what I wanted from the rest of my life. I refused to even *consider* the possibility of a Plan B or the idea that a life without children, might, in the end, suit me just fine. It was a heresy and I swear that writing it right now still makes me feel nauseous and ashamed. That's the taboo in action, even now, rumbling on in my subconscious.

Because it didn't occur to me that a life without children was possible, I never gave it any energy – which means that I never really put any energy into the life I was *actually living*. No wonder it was a mess. I starved my lived reality of life force and then I wondered why it felt like I was dying inside…

THE DARK SIDE OF DAYDREAMS

I think of the 'shadow life' as the life you dreamt about while your 'real life' was happening and to which you gave so much energy that it depleted the life you were *actually* living. I see it as the shadow of the life unlived.

I'm not saying that dreaming about motherhood was wrong; it's perhaps just the *amount* of energy you invested in those daydreams that was unbalanced.

> When your daydreams are sucking the life force out of your lived life, you've sprung a psychic leak!

Letting go of your shadow life means first that you have to bring it into the light of your awareness and take a good look at it. This can be quite scary because it's a bit like waking up and trying to put a dream into words and feeling the 'meaning' of your dream slip away. What felt magical becomes prosaic and you feel the loss. It seems safer to keep it all to yourself.

Doing this will also probably bring more grief to the surface, but perhaps you might be ready to see that as more healing rather than as a signal to repress those thoughts, those feelings.

If, in your shadow life as a mother, you imagined a loving partner and playing in the garden with your children, whilst in your real life you were both single and living in an apartment with a window-box full of dead plants, there's a kind of disconnection between these two that doesn't feel great. When you bring it into the light, it can stir up feelings of anger, bitterness, blame, depression and resentfulness. This is a natural part of grief, and letting go is what grief is all about.

Hanging onto an old dream takes a lot of energy – energy that could be better used making a new, maybe even better life come into being.

> Letting go of daydreams is hard because, frankly,
> letting go of anything is hard!

When I was still hopeful of having a child and completely in denial about the reality of my situation, I felt I couldn't change the reel in my personal dream cinema because, if I did, maybe I was being disloyal to my dreams of becoming a mother. I think at some deep level I understood that this dream was sucking the life out of me but I refused to allow it to evolve as my life took a different direction. The kind of self-reflective analysis I would apply to any other area of my life, I withheld from this sacred part of myself. I was too scared to look closely because it felt like the 'dream' was all I had left.

Letting go of my dream of motherhood felt like letting go of that very last part of me that *was* a mother. I fought it like hell. But once I was ready, it wasn't nearly as bad as I expected. Now, at night, I don't dream of babies anymore. Not flying babies, not being pregnant, not of a little girl holding my hand. I dream of other things, new things.

You can't force this stage because truly letting go of this dream is a major loss. We're losing our family. Only you'll know when you're ready to let go of the string and let this fantasy balloon float away...

GETTING TO KNOW YOUR SHADOW LIFE

Each of us who wanted to become a mother has our own themes and storylines in our shadow story, but here are some that you might recognise in yours.

- **The Happy Family Fantasy**

  For many of us, what we craved was not just a baby, but a family. We wanted to be part of something, to create something bigger than ourselves. Yes, we craved the unconditional love of an infant, but we also wanted a partner and siblings in the picture. We saw ourselves in the kitchen, at family gatherings. Perhaps you had a snapshot in your mind of a perfect little family, like the iconic families used by advertising to sell us stuff? But ask yourself this – weren't we perhaps being a little unreasonable expecting our family to turn out perfectly? Do you actually know any perfect families? Is your own family of origin perfect? Like all 'shadow life' vignettes, there's nothing weird about this except perhaps you might like to wonder if part of your longing for a perfect family was in some way driven by a need to right the wrongs of your own childhood and to finally satisfy your own unmet childhood needs. Did you want to make the family you never had? Was perhaps the little girl in you, one of your Russian dolls, running the projector for this emotional film? I imagine that this is a perfectly normal and healthy desire, but it is yet one more loss we have to metabolise – that we will never get the chance to right the wrongs of our own upbringing by doing things differently with our own children.

- **The Perfect Mother Fantasy**

  Each of us has a different idea of what kind of 'Perfect Mother' we were going to be: mine was a sort of skinny rock-chick in faded Levi 501s and a white t-shirt with long hair flowing down her lean back, no make-up, a light tan with a smattering of freckles and a cute baby on her hip. This fantasy takes place in a huge country-meets-city kitchen full of wonderful smells, intelligent talk radio burbling in the background, the book I've just published in view and a cute mop-headed four-year-old at the kitchen table making naïve yet insightful remarks.

This fantasy persisted despite the fact that I'm not naturally skinny and haven't been so for a decade now and that far from looking elegant without make up I probably would have been looking shattered from lack of sleep (I'm a poor sleeper as it is!) Let alone the inconvenient fact that it's proving hard enough to find the time to finish this book *without* children! And, in reality, a four-year old with a new sibling would be more likely to be singing inane nursery rhymes over and over again until I wanted to scream with frustration, whilst looking for ways to poke a stick in the new baby's eye when my back was turned! But reality? I had no use for it.

- **The Perfect Children Fantasy**

I'm not sure about you, but my shadow life rarely featured a stroppy teenager, a kid on drugs, a two-year-old having a tantrum or a child with learning difficulties or other challenges. It was always some version of the Partridge Family or the Waltons but with a British twist. I could see how 'my' baby would fit into 'my' dream, but in truth that baby was an extension of my dreams of motherhood. In my Perfect Children Fantasy I'd get on brilliantly with my kids because we'd have similar personalities, aspirations and talents – although they'd be good at maths, which I'm not.

This is about as realistic as Disney. But bringing my shadow family into the light meant looking at the reality of being a mother married to an irresponsible artist and chaotic alcoholic whilst trying to run a business, hold a marriage together, and bring up children. A lot more like reality TV and a lot less like the Partridge Family. My dreams were just that, 'my dreams' and my child would have had 'their dreams' which no doubt would have been completely different. If I'd had children, my daughter might have turned out to be a TV-obsessed princess fascinated by make-up and status, whilst my son could have been a non-academic football-mad boy who just wanted to play sport and violent video games. That tomboy daughter with a love of nature, books and the unseen world? A mini me. That creative, delicate and brilliant son? A mini him of my husband. In truth, I was playing dollies in my mind; it was fun but it came at a high cost to the life I was actually living.

DEMOLISHING THE WENDY HOUSE

You may never have doubted for a moment that you wanted to become a mother. You may have played with dolls as a child, had names for your children picked out before you were ten years old and known that being a mother was part of your destiny for as long as you can remember. Or you may not have. I didn't.

Looking back on my own childhood games in the Wendy house (or whatever the name might have been of any make believe 'house' you played in as a girl), it was never about being a mother. It was about independence and being in charge.

I know that I made a decision when I was very young that when I grew up I was *never* going to get married and have children. But this wasn't a decision, nor even a free choice really – rather it was a reaction to my own mother's unhappiness. It was also, at a deeper level, somewhere to 'put' my own unhappiness and confusion as a child. Although I couldn't have told you this until my 40s, the reason I didn't think I wanted children until I was almost 30 was because I was terrified that 'having a child' meant revisiting the darker moments of my childhood. And also, subconsciously, I feared that having been brought up by a mother who was still struggling with the wounds of her *own* childhood, I wouldn't really be up to the job.

Ambivalence about Motherhood

Ambivalence about becoming a mother is quite natural. After all, it's a huge risk, a gamble and a lifelong one at that. It's not something you can ever change your mind about. We need to remember that it's only been just over 50 years since the pill became widely available[43] after hundreds of thousands of years of sex meaning a strong possibility of having a child. Making a conscious decision to *stop* contraception and become a mother is not something that women have yet had much psychological experience with – and it's a decision that we can't entirely rely on logic and common sense to make. We want to be sure that it's a good idea, but there are no assurances it will be. All we can be sure of is that whatever the outcome is, there's no turning back. All other big life decisions, including with whom to form a life-long partnership, can be revised. But if motherhood turns out not to be right for you – tough. You can give your child up for adoption, but that doesn't mean that you're no longer a mother: you're a mother who gave up her child, and that's another taboo too, being a 'bad mother'.

There are some women who are so certain from a very young age that they are childfree by choice and that they will *never* want children that they seek medical sterilisation in their twenties, but often have a very hard time finding a surgeon who will agree to do so. The idea that they are bound to change their minds 'one day' is so entrenched in our culture that doctors don't want to take the risk of depriving them of children at a later date. It seems that our pronatalist culture literally can't 'conceive' of a woman who is absolutely sure that she doesn't want children – considering her to be, in some profound way, 'unnatural'.

As a childless-by-circumstance woman, I sometimes answer the 'Why don't you have kids?' question with, 'I couldn't' which, although it's only part of the story, is usually enough information. But if your answer is, 'I didn't want them' it's frequently a whole different conversation, mainly because the prejudices that some people have about childless women, but which they don't say to our faces, are often freely spoken to childfree women. Statements such as, 'But you won't know what it is to be a woman until you've given birth,' or 'Isn't that rather selfish?' or 'Who's going to look after you when you're old? – you'll regret it then!'

The pronatalist belief that it is every woman's destiny to become a mother plays out differently in the lives of childfree and childless women. However, surely it is much better that women who are *absolutely sure* they don't want children can honour that self-awareness rather than end up as reluctant mothers? Perhaps our culture's abhorrence of their 'unnaturalness' or 'selfishness' says more about many people's fear of not fitting in than it does about *their* self-awareness and self-definition?

The Non-Decision that Becomes a Decision

Unrecognised ambivalence, which often 'hides' in the deferral of a decision about motherhood until it's a non-decision which becomes a decision, appears to be a common experience for women who find themselves childless in their 40s and can't quite work out how it happened. Having convinced themselves that a baby was something that was 'just going to happen' or that 'the right person was just going to come along', or that 'they'd conceive when the time was right' they remained in denial about the approaching end to their fertility.

However, if they tried to express their '3am thoughts' (as I often refer to them, and women usually nod in recognition) usually all they'd hear back from others would be echoes of, 'Don't worry, the right person will come along', 'Just relax', or some other version of a miracle baby story or fairytale ending.

Many women move into their 30s confident that this is the decade they'll become mothers but, due to circumstances outside their control, or which they *decide* are out of their control (jobs, relationships, health, money, housing, fertility, economy, parental illness, etc) it doesn't happen and doesn't happen and still doesn't happen. As they are, at some deep level, fundamentally unclear about whether they really want a baby or not, they let 'the universe' decide for them. But 'the universe' mirrors back to them their own ambivalence, and so it remains unclear. (Deferring to 'the universe' is the latest get-out-of-jail-free card for really sticky decisions). And then as their 40s loom on the horizon they realise, with a shock, that they're running out of time and often start making frantic efforts to have a baby before it's too late and get so caught up in the dynamics of panic that they *still* don't take the time to get to the bottom of their ambivalence. Babymania takes over from ambivalence and the roots of those feelings remain unexplored. The panicky mantra seems to be, 'What if I really *do* want a child and I don't find out until it's too late?'

For some, this mad dash ends with a baby. For others it doesn't. But the ambivalence over becoming a mother goes underground as a taboo once you've had a child. Mothers, you see, aren't 'allowed' to wonder if having children was a good idea, although many of them do. In a 'National Parenting Survey' conducted by Oprah's Dr Phil in 2003 with over 20,000 respondents, 40% of parents said that if they knew then what they knew now, they wouldn't make the same choice.[44] According to Laura Carroll, 'anonymous surveys of parents have shown even higher percentages'.[45]

One of my childfree-by-choice friends tells me that when she explains her choice to mothers, they frequently 'confess' (their word) to her that, if they had their time again, they wouldn't have had their children either. Much as they love them, they've come to realise that 'motherhood's not what they thought it would be', that they've 'lost their identity' and that they've become 'invisible'. Such things are taboo to say to anyone who isn't a mother because it makes them sound like they don't love their children, which isn't the case. Life isn't that simple: mothers can love their children and still regret taking on the grinding, relentless domestic tasks of motherhood – but that human, nuanced complexity, that's lost in our pronatalist society. Mothers know it, and they share this 'dark secret' with each other – they're just not allowed to tell 'anyone else'. Their current social script reads, 'It's the most fulfilling thing I've ever done', just as ours reads, 'I'll never get over not being a mother.' But life isn't that predictable.

For those last-dashers who *don't* end up with a baby, our unexplored ambivalence becomes yet another stick with which to beat ourselves up – we tell ourselves that because we didn't *really* want a baby it didn't happen. But this is a kind of magical thinking – telling ourselves that if we'd wanted a baby 'harder' it would have worked out differently. We think that if we'd been clearer in our desires when we were younger we would have made different decisions. There's some truth in that, but it's a bitter truth and a pointless one because we can't go back and do it differently. And I also know plenty of women who've been very, very sure from a very early age of their desire to become mothers, and it hasn't worked out for them either. How can you tell a woman who's endured multiple rounds of IVF that she obviously didn't *really* want children? The fact is, there are no guarantees that we get what we want in life despite what our consumer culture tells us. And don't get me started on the kind of magical thinking promoted by books like 'The Secret' and which the fertility industry has latched onto as a marketing tool par excellence. Grrrrrr.

The Gifts of Ambivalence

There's nothing wrong with us if we were ambivalent about having children. I'll repeat that, because it's so important:

> There's nothing wrong with us if we were ambivalent about having children.

Ambivalence shows that, at some deep level, we were truly considering the reality of parenting and whether or not it was the kind of lifelong commitment we could really cope with or be good at. We were thinking of our unborn children's lives as well as our own. Ambivalence about having children is intelligence and compassion in action. It does not mean we were not fit to be mothers, no matter what you've convinced yourself and however it affected the decisions and non-decisions that contributed to your childlessness.

Within your ambivalence may be the seeds of your recovery from an unhappily childless life. Having those thoughts meant that you were, to some degree, conscious that there were *other* possibilities for you in life other than becoming a mother. Having those thoughts may have felt disloyal to your dream, but now that you're looking to get your Plan B going, they may well blossom into a meaningful and fulfilling life without children.

If we begin to explore our ambivalence for the options that we worried about giving up, we will begin to find its gifts. It's time to stop feeling guilty about our ambivalence and instead to celebrate our ability to dream alternative dreams.

For millennia there have been women who have had dreams other than the dream of motherhood and it has been impossible for them to fulfil them. Once we put down the unholy trinity of guilt, shame and blame, we too can start to live out other dreams of how to be a woman in this world.

Exercise 8: Declutter Your Dreams

Imagine that you are writing a letter or email to an old friend that you've been out of touch with since schooldays. In this email, you're filling them in on your story since then and telling them all about your children and daily life.

Write it in the present tense as if it were true. Describe your partner, your kids, what they're like, what your life is like. Try not to edit this fantasy with your rational mind but allow yourself to indulge in it to its full extent. Make it as vivid and detail-rich as you can. This is the last time you're going to do this, so go for it.

Now, create a ritual to help you let it go. If you have another Gateway Woman who can be with you and witness your ceremony, or if you can do it together, you'll find it a powerfully supportive experience.

Go to a private place that is special or sacred to you. When you're ready, read your letter out loud and then choose a way in which to let it go. You might like to burn it, rip it up into tiny pieces and let the wind take it, bury it in the earth or put it into flowing water like a stream or the ocean. Whatever feels right to you and has the beauty and symbolism you need. Say any prayers or wishes that feel appropriate to you. You might want to read a poem, play some music or sing a special song.

Even if this feels like a silly idea, please honour your dream of motherhood by letting it go with love and ritual. Our culture has become devoid of rituals apart from marriage, parenting and death, but it's a deep human need and we are a poorer culture for having lost so many of them. And as childless-by-circumstance women we are each painfully aware that we miss out on the milestones and rituals of family life – so our need for this ritual is all the greater.

By creating this ritual of letting go, you are honouring yourself and the family you dreamt of having.

If you have any keepsakes or baby clothes or anything that you've been saving for your children, now might be the time to think of passing them on to someone who can use them. If you have a book or folder on your computer with possible baby names, it's time to let those go too, along with any information you were keeping about IVF, any leftover drugs or paraphernalia and anything else that you know was related to your dream of motherhood. Only you will know what to keep and what to let go of at this time, so trust yourself and if there's something you can't bear to be parted from just yet, keep it, and revisit this exercise in a year's time.

Just as we need to declutter our life, we need to declutter our dreams. Without letting go, there can be no space in our life and heart for a new dream. It's time to let go. Let go with love.

Reflections on this Chapter

In this chapter we've looked at some of the fantasies we've been holding onto about the family we longed to have and how perfect it would have been. We've also begun exploring how our own childhood may have influenced our decisions about motherhood, and how those ideas may have fed into any ambivalence we felt about becoming mothers in the first place.

Beginning to lift the lid on parts of our life that we may not have thought about for a long time can be quite painful. As you've probably worked out by now, it's not an excuse to beat yourself up. You're building up a detailed picture of how and why you got to where you are today not so that you have more ammunition to prove how dumb you've been, but rather to understand things more fully. Because, buried in the dark, hidden in those places that we don't want to look are also the very things we need to dig out, polish up and bring into the light of our new lives. As Jung said, 'The gold is in the dark'.

If you did the 'Declutter Your Dreams' exercise then you have my deepest respect – it takes a lot of courage – but I hope this moving and powerful way to shift things has opened a part of your heart that may have been shut for a long time. And if you didn't do it, please consider doing it at a later date, when you feel ready. The reason that all human cultures have rituals is that their symbolism makes visible the invisible transitions from one stage of our lives to another. Your dreams of a family may have been such a big part of your life that their passing deserves to be honoured with tenderness and witnessed with respect as you move to the next stage of your life. As do you.

You don't have a body;
you are a body.

CHAPTER 8

RECONNECTING TO YOUR SOURCE

How Your Recovery from Childlessness Affects Your Relationships with Yourself and Others

Perhaps only other women who have experienced involuntary childlessness can comprehend how absolutely and completely betrayed by life some of us can feel. I sometimes imagine that mothers who tragically lose a child may experience a similar loss, but one so much more visceral than ours. I know that some of us envy the fact that at least they have 'someone' to mourn, that their grief and loss is culturally recognised and that they know what it is to be a mother. It is an identity that can never be taken from them, painful as it is. But spare a thought for the fact that they too are expected to 'get over it' as if it were flu, a heartlessness which I could never have imagined, but which many bereaved mothers have since told me about.

To be childless, when for many years you may have reserved a place in your heart, soul and life for a family, is a loss that's hard for others to comprehend. Sometimes, I wonder what it would have been like to have known since childhood that having children was impossible – as it is for those who are born without a womb or have conditions diagnosed in puberty that mean they will never be fertile. I fantasised that, had that been the case for me, that I wouldn't have shaped such a huge chunk of my adult hopes around becoming a mother. But then as I've got to know women for whom this is their reality, I've heard heartbreaking stories of how challenging it can be to become 'a woman' when you know you will never be able to get pregnant naturally, so wrapped up is motherhood with the identity of womanhood.

> At some deep level, part of the devastation of childlessness is that we feel a profound sense of being betrayed by life, by our bodies and by ourselves.

The shift in identity from being a woman who hopes, one day, to become a mother to one who knows, without question, that it's never going to happen is so huge that it throws *everything* into question. This life-changing threshold is invisible to others and, as yet, little understood or spoken about – but those of us living through it know that it's perhaps the toughest challenge we've faced so far.

We may be dealing with a deep sense of betrayal of ourselves by ourselves, and this can lead us to question the very nature of our relationship with ourselves, our bodies and our belief systems. Those who haven't experienced this accuse me of exaggerating how it feels but I'm not. These are our truths and sometimes they are extreme.

During this process of questioning everything, perhaps unsure about who we are any more and in the process of re-examining the nature of our relationship with ourselves, we may also find that every other single relationship in our life comes under scrutiny. This next little exercise will hopefully help to show why that is.

EXERCISE 9: GOING DOTTY

Either do this in your imagination or grab a bit of paper.

Imagine all the relationships in your life as a sort of 'map' made up of 'dots'. You are a dot at the centre and around you, also represented by dots, are your key relationships – your partner, family, friends, colleagues, etc. If you draw a line between your dot and each of the other dots, each line will be a different length and at a different angle to you.

Now, imagine that you move the dot representing you to a different place – even by the tiniest amount. See what happens to the lines?

By moving yourself, even a tiny amount, you are at a different angle and distance from absolutely everyone else in your life.

So, along with the internal change we're dealing with, it may seem like we also have to deal with what can feel like an endless amount of change in *all* our relationships. Think of it like a life renegotiation – you're not the same person you were when you made the 'deals' that form your current relationship patterns and so for you to move forward, they're all up for renegotiation. Whether you, or they, like it or not.

This can be incredibly hard on those around us. Because what *they* thought and felt was secure and a 'done deal' is now being renegotiated, it might seem pretty unfair to them. After all, not only have they supported you through some of the most difficult years of your life, but now that you're coming out the other side there's a whole new set of problems to be got through. But that's life – always on the move, always changing. When a plant stops growing, it dies. So do we, in subtle ways.

The process of healing from loss is a process of change. I imagine it as an expansion of our identity until it's big enough to include and integrate that loss. Grieving changes us and we are never the same again after loving someone or grieving someone.

When couples lose a child, the impact of that bereavement can break up the relationship. When one partner in a relationship goes into recovery (from alcoholism for example) it too can often lead to a relationship breakdown. And for couples who are coming to terms with the end of their 'trying-to-conceive' journey or who have suffered miscarriage, early term loss and stillbirth, or perhaps are trying to move forward without children because one partner has changed their mind about having children or for any of the many, many reasons we find ourselves without the child we expected, this loss can become a major stumbling block to continued connection.

Such losses, so huge to process, may become so difficult to talk about that they become a block in the relationship and perhaps, in the end, it may seem easier to split up than to work out what to do about the 'baby elephant in the room'.

Intimacy and honesty are, in fact, the same thing.

Faced with this, couples may turn away from each other or enter into a 'pretend' intimacy – a sort of *intimacy-lite* – which doesn't fool either of them for long, but may be thought of perhaps as the 'denial' stage of their grieving process as a couple. For many couples, the necessary 'anger' stage of grief is one that they don't feel able to deal with together – or conversely they may be so angry that they destroy the relationship by taking it out on each other. In order to do our grief work *within* our relationship we will need support *from outside* our primary relationship.

As well as our relationship with our partner (if we have one), our relationships with family, friends and colleagues also come in for a bashing. Now that you've officially either 'given up trying' or have made some kind of public declaration that you've accepted that it's not going to happen for you, people may well breathe a big sigh of relief and expect things to 'get back to normal'.

But there is no 'normal' to go back to. I spent 15 years of my life longing to be a mother, giving up hope at 43½ that it was not to be and falling headfirst into my grieving process. But even the fact that I'd given up didn't stop people continuing to bombard me with miracle baby stories and they still do. These days it's more often the 'Why don't you just adopt?' comment (don't you just love that 'just'!) rather than the 'Don't give up, you never know, it's never too late' – but they're not based in any reality. It doesn't seem to occur to them that as a single working woman I have neither the time nor the financial resources to adopt internationally, and that as someone who has written publicly about her grief and depression over childlessness I would not be considered a suitable candidate for a domestic adoption. I've also lost count of the number of financially and emotionally stable childless couples I know of who've been turned down as adoptive parents, or who've been approved, but after years of waiting for a match have given up. There's only so much hope and heartbreak you can live with before you realise that your sanity is hanging on by a thread. As one infertile woman I know puts it when she and her husband are asked why they haven't adopted, 'We maxed out the heartbreak cards already'.

The reality is that surviving and thriving after childlessness changes every aspect of our life and relationships. Colleagues who may have relied upon us to be the one they turned to when they were having a difficult day may find that we're no longer quite the pushover for a sob story we once were. Siblings who've expected us to be their free unpaid babysitter for life may be confused when we develop other priorities. Friends may find our new energy and commitment to things that they're not interested in (or don't have the time for as parents) confronting and difficult. And our partners may not know who we are anymore. And we're not sure yet, either.

Coming to terms with our childlessness as a permanent identity is a shift that changes everything and everyone around us. It's important to recognise that and to be understanding of other people's reactions and to make allowances for them, if possible. Some of our relationships may dissolve as we grow and change and find new relationships that suit us better. Some relationships will evolve along with us.

The fact is not everyone *wants* to be as free of illusion and as emotionally and psychologically mature as we are becoming. And it's neither our right nor our job to tell them that they need to. There's also no need to jettison relationships that don't seem to be working anymore as part of the emotional house-clearance you may be embarking upon. It may well be that although we're moving 'away' from those people at the moment, part of our healing might be that we are travelling in a very big spiral and that it's a relationship we'll be grateful for again one day.

Some Tips:

- Be gentle with yourself and others throughout this process of relationship renegotiation.

- Learning to actively practise self-compassion will help you, and others, deal with the changes. (More on that in Chapter 9)

- Be honest about what you're going through and ask for patience and tolerance from others, and give it back twice over. Childlessness is a taboo and others may be scared and uncomfortable around us – educate them how to support you rather than expecting them to be mind readers.

- Stop expecting others to understand your situation. In answer to a question I put to Brené Brown at a public talk in July 2013[46], infertility and childlessness has shown up in her research as 'the number one area of empathy failure'. Your friends and family are not *uniquely* clueless!

- Recognise that you don't yet know who you're becoming – you're a work in progress. Try not to make any irrevocable decisions for a couple of years at least. Grieving changes us in surprising (and often wonderful) ways.

- Understand that your grieving and healing affects everyone and everything around you. Even if you're *not* talking about it, it has a shape and presence that can be challenging for others to cope with as it may bring *their* ungrieved losses to the surface.

- Accept that no one else will change to your timetable. No one. Even if they promise they will. Give it up and focus on your own healing.

- It's OK to 'park' a friendship or relationship if it's too hot to deal with right now – you don't need to be an emotional ninja… Sometimes a 'cooling off' period works for everyone and once you feel a bit clearer about things you (and they) can take it from there.

- Get support from outside your primary relationships and give the people in your intimate circle a rest from your issues – this is when the sisterhood of other childless-by-circumstance women can be so powerful.

Time to Stop Punishing Yourself

Living with a body that we felt was 'meant' to have children can be hard once that dream is over. Sometimes it's easier to disconnect from it altogether after all we've been through.

- We may have put our bodies through hellish medical procedures in the hopes of having a baby, only to end up with empty bank accounts, broken bodies and broken dreams.

- We may have made ourselves sick with hope, that most toxic of fertility drugs.
- We may have endured miscarriages and early-term loss or we may never have got pregnant.
- We may have nurtured our bodies through decades of menstruation – been disciplined and honourable with our birth control, taken vitamins, kept fit, eaten a healthy diet and treated ourselves as mothers-to-be – only to never even have had a *chance* to try for a baby. We may feel at the bottom of the pile of childless-by-circumstance women, judging ourselves on some invisible pecking order of shame and deny ourselves even the right to feel *included* in the collective pain of childless women.

And these days, now that we know we will never be mothers, we may be ignoring our body altogether to the point of neglect.

> What's the point of these breasts if they will never feed a child? This rounded belly if it will never keep a growing baby safe? These hips if they were never meant for childbirth? What's the point of this womanly body at all?

We may be at the beginnings of peri-menopause or menopausal – our skin, hair and hormones reminding us that our girlish days are well and truly behind us. The periods that tied us to the rhythm of the moon, like the mysterious creatures we are, now quieting, or flooding, or silent. The river gone still, underground. We may be living in our heads these days – staying late at work when we don't really need to, numbing out by watching too much TV, mindlessly checking Facebook and wandering around our homes as if we're looking for something that we left somewhere, but just can't quite remember what it is, or where we put it.

We have lost our connection to source.

Our body is our spirit made flesh. Whatever your faith or whether you have no faith, if you wanted to have a child you know that there is something sacred about a woman's body and its ability to bring forth life and you feel denied *your* part in that sacrament.

> But you were a sacred birth once. You are still sacred.

By blaming our body we internalise the shame and rage we feel about how things have worked out for us; we bury it alive in our flesh. We wall ourselves in with it. It is easier to grab the flesh on our hips and say, 'I'm disgusting' than it is to feel the grief contained in our lost hopes for those curves, that womanly fat.

It is easier to stop caring about our bodies, eating rubbish food and never taking any exercise, than it is to work through our sense of having failed and being unable to imagine a future that fills us with any sense of hope or excitement.

It's easier to deny ourselves bodily pleasure, to withdraw from the body, to withdraw from sex with our partner (or find it hard to enjoy it as we once did), to give up looking for a relationship and resign ourselves to celibacy, to starve and over-exercise as a way of punishing ourselves, than it is to feel the pain of our crushing betrayal by life.

Our body is sacred, but *we* don't feel worthy of that sacrament anymore.

Forgiving Your Body

Forgiving our body is forgiving ourself for getting it wrong, for failing, for every 'stupid' decision we made that got us to the place we are today. For the illnesses and inheritances that made it too difficult or impossible to have a baby. For the wanderings and wonderings of our early womanhood whilst we tried to work out who we were, before we could even think about becoming mothers.

We need our bodies to have that future – we're not going to get there by thought alone! But we can't dump so much of the pain from our unmet longings into our flesh and then expect it to spring into action, reborn, revitalised and ready to go once we're ready to move towards our Plan B. Our body is not a tool, there to carry out our wishes; it *is* our wishes. Every thought, every dream, every experience is written on our body, in our body.

> Forgiving our body is an act of grace that frees us up to start imagining that we have a future again. That we *deserve* a future again.

It has been said that 'we are not human beings having a spiritual experience – we are spiritual beings having a human experience'.[47] The fact is, however you look at it, the 'you' that is reading this book is bigger than this body, these mistakes, these unlucky breaks, this heartbreak. And thus you can transcend and transform this pain into a new and passionate life. This is the gift of being both spirit and body, yoked by a creative mind.

But first, you have to forgive your body.

Deep down, we know that there's healing to be done. And we fear that healing as much as we long for it. In Chapter 4 we started exploring our grief around our childlessness and letting that process of healing move through us.

Now we also need to mourn our youth, our strength, our fertility. There is more to us than these bodies, but we can't do anything without them. However much you want to deny that you have a body, however much you want to punish it, it's not going to go away.

Yes, you are more than that, but as long as you deny your body the love it craves, you are denying yourself the support you need to move forward. You can't drag your body with you, reluctantly. You've got to make this trip together, willingly.

Hating your body, hating yourself won't make things better; it will make them worse. Allowing yourself to grieve the losses your body has lived through with you will allow it to heal, and as it heals, you heal. As you change, your body changes with you. Because your body *is* you.

> Because you don't have a body; you are a body.

Learning to Love Your Body Again

Right now, you may be wondering what the hell I'm on about – *Has she gone all beardy-weirdy on me now?* But this idea that our bodies *are* us, not some machine that we control, strikes at the very heart of the mind-body duality that has dominated Western thinking since the Enlightenment. Science, the astonishing product of Enlightenment thinking is beginning, with its explorations into quantum realms, to accept the idea that there is an intelligence at work in our bodies and in the universe which is non-rational and immensely smart. And perhaps even non-local in some instances too.

We are not dumb flesh run by a smart computer. We are spirit (intelligence if you prefer) made flesh – and way smarter than the smartest computer. Forgiving our bodies is not mere lip service to some new-age touchy-feely idea. It has immense power.

Is it not a contradiction that many of us see our bodies as instruments of our mind and as tools to carry out our wishes and yet, when our goal is self-destruction and our tool is neglect, we get angry with our bodies for following our instructions to the letter?

Loving your body is an act of profound acceptance and healing that will strengthen and support you as you learn to cherish yourself and your life again. I'm not suggesting the kind of regime that you might find in a women's magazine, but rather a conscious decision to offer gratitude to your body for getting you this far and a willingness to be grateful to it in the future. If this body had borne children, flesh of your flesh, how tenderly would you regard the flesh of your children?

> It's time to stop denying yourself the love you deserve.
> It is the same flesh that your children would have been made of.

The body that you love and feel at home in already exists. You don't have to create it by your own will. It is there, you just have to remember it and then find your way back to it.

There is a place in your memory, I hope, of a time when you were a young girl before you divorced yourself from your body – when you and your flesh moved and thought and felt and dreamt as one. For me, it is a memory of standing ankle-high in a babbling brook with a butterfly net in my hand, fishing for the tiny stickleback fish darting around the rocks. The sun is on my back and dancing on the water, whilst the shadow of the footbridge lies dark and cool behind me. I am totally absorbed in the bright, laughing water and my body moves with me like a silent wriggling fish. We are one.

This union is our birthright yet our culture, wonderful in so many ways, has also created a glory in the artificial, the easy to spot, the flashy. But these moments of poise and stillness when our spirit and body breathe together and know each other to be true, this honest joining is the kind of bodily integrity on which new dreams can be built.

Finding Your Source

Each of us, regardless of our beliefs, lack of beliefs, religious views and observances or not, has to find a way back to source.

What is source?

It is the endless boundlessness of our spirit, our intelligence, our essential self. You don't have to believe that it goes on after your death – you don't have to believe anything anyone else tells you. But I would like to invite you to believe that you are more than your childlessness.

And to do that, you need to stop, be quiet and listen to your body and to the sweet simplicity of your nature under all your negative beliefs and broken dreams.

There is a space at the core of us all; a deep pool of quietness filled with love. It took me a long time to connect with it after the knocks and disasters of life, but when I found my way back there, I realised that I was home again. Moreover, after a while, I came to understand that it is not a *place* at all where I go. I am already there. It *is* me, and I am it. It is a boundless place of freedom, curiosity, joy and compassion and when I was a child I knew it as intimately as the scene from my bedroom window. But then I learned about school things and all the ways that I was 'wrong', and I lost contact with my underground river, my essential self, my source.

The contemplative part of all religions and philosophies comes from this place, from source. Most of us become gradually disconnected from it at some point in our youth, and although many of us may continue to have faith of some kind and perhaps may even be observant of that faith, few of us remain in daily contact with the source of that faith. You don't have to believe in anything to have access to source; it runs through everything and everyone and is our birthright. We are all made of the same material that fires the sun and unfurls the buds of spring. We are all made of source; we are all part of source.

> Creativity comes from source; love comes from source; compassion comes from source; forgiveness comes from source; hope and resilience come from source. We come from source. We are source.

If we are to open ourselves up to the possibility of a meaningful and fulfilling life without children, we need to connect to source in a way that works for us, as often as we can. I recommend daily.

We are *massively* going against the grain of our culture by daring to give birth to ourselves anew as a way to recover from our childlessness.

It is an act of colossal courage and given little regard, respect or credence by most others. There is very little support, hardly any recognition and no award ceremonies for remaking our lives around a new core of meaning. As I've said before, no one really gives a damn what we do with our lives now as long as we pay our taxes, keep quiet and take care of sick and elderly relatives. Because of this, we need to gather our support for the changes we're going through from a deeper place and from each other.

Even our partners, family and closest friends may disagree or ridicule what we're trying to do. The fact is, when someone, anyone, chooses to consciously heal, this can be very challenging for those around them. Because as we heal, it touches the desire in *them* to heal – and rather than it inspiring them, they may feel guilty about their own resistance and project that back onto us as hostility, cynicism and ridicule.

So, expect some flak from others as you begin to change. In fact, you might find that it's better to keep quiet about what you're up to in the early stages, when it's so easy to be knocked off course by an unsupportive or critical remark from someone we care about. Instead, seek the support of people interested and active on a path of personal transformation and if they're also childless women, all the better!

> You don't need to convert anyone, or convince anyone.
> Just do your thing, and shine.

The support of other childless-by-circumstance women and a connection to source is, in my experience, vital to get your healing project on the road. In time, others will want what you've got, but until you've got it, they're unlikely to give you any help or support to get it! No one believes a prophet in their own land. Keep quiet and let others notice how 'well you're looking these days', how much 'happier' or 'calmer' you seem.

Each of us connects to source in our own way and it might take a bit of experimentation to find the way that works for you and is sustainable. It's all very well going away on a meditation retreat and feeling all pure and 'spiritual' on the journey home, but if you can't fit it around your day-to-day life, it's not a reliable way for you to connect to source.

Opening Up Your Connection to Source

Here are some suggestions taken from my own experience from years of reading, experimenting, failing, starting again, giving up, losing heart and somehow managing to keep on going. More information in the 'Recommended Reading' section of the Appendix if you want to explore further:

- Give up reading women's magazines and watching TV that promotes the idea that your body is something to be perfected. Unplug from the toxic crap that makes you feel 'less than' (that includes a lot of social media too). Consume media intelligently and compassionately – would you have let your kids get their values this way? Thought not.

- Do Julia Cameron's 'Morning Pages' exercise from her book, The Artist's Way.[48]

- Attend 12 Step meetings of any kind. These are usually called *Something* Anonymous, with the most famous one being Alcoholics Anonymous. However, there are meetings for all kinds of issues, including DA (Debtors Anonymous) which is for anyone with a cranky relationship with money – and as money and self-worth are closely aligned, it's really enlightening.

- Make something: writing, blogging, painting, gardening, engine building, homemaking, singing, baking, sewing, tap-dancing…

- Take a walk alone in nature (woods and hills do it for me, but for you it might be the sea, or arid plains…)

- Try meditating (not as hard as it sounds). There are even phone apps to help you get into the habit.

- Practice self-compassion. I recommend Kristin Neff's book 'Self Compassion'[49] to understand the power of this approach and why it's very different from selfishness or self-obsession.

- Give up perfectionism and embrace mistakes, failure, bloopers and getting it wrong as part of being human. Brené Brown's my heroine on this one – read 'The Gifts of Imperfection'[50] to understand why.

- Find a way to touch the sublime: great architecture, sacred buildings, inspiring art, an astonishing film, poetry. Anything that touches your soul and fills you with a sense of awe – of expansiveness.

- Take some exercise: for me the best are yoga, walking, swimming and cycling. But for you it might be football, skydiving and croquet!

- Listen to pure birdsong recordings, without any annoying plinkity-plonkity new age music. I've found that British and European sounds work best for me; you might find that a recording from the environment you grew up in as a very young girl has a special quality for you too.

- Speak up in the face of abuse, unkindness or injustice. There's nothing like giving my inner warrior an outlet to connect me to a place of power and truth.

- Do acts of random kindness and thoughtfulness. Read Mike Dickson's inspiring book 'Please Take One'[51] on the power of generosity for inspiration.

- Live from a place of integrity, especially when no one is looking.

- Seek out inspirational and spiritual literature from different faiths and traditions.

- Watch TED.com videos of inspirational talks

- Choose to spend time around people who inspire you, make you laugh, remind you of the best of you and who support you on the path towards your Plan B.

Exercise 10: Saying Thank You

The next time you take a shower or bath, take a moment to say 'thank you' to each part of your body as you lovingly wash it. This simple act of treating your body with respect and gratitude can release a lot of repressed emotion and memories.

Allow the tears to come or the anger, shame or whatever it is that arises, and let the water wash it away. Let the stuck emotion flow and be gentle and tender towards yourself as it does. Imagine that you are 'little you' or the child you wished you had given birth to and treat yourself with gentleness, love and respect. No judgement, no recrimination, no 'I shouldn't be feeling this'. If you're feeling it, you're feeling it – it really is that simple.

Afterwards, dry yourself tenderly and take the time to moisturise your skin, paying particular attention to any parts you may have disliked or blamed in the past.

Remain really present and try not to drift away into your head – I like to say *thank you* to each part of my body in turn in a specific way – it looks a bit crazy when I write it down but I'll say thank you to my elbows 'for being so flexible', to my back 'for standing up for me' and so on and so on. After you've finished this exercise you will hopefully find that your whole body is zinging with energy and that you have a warm glow inside you. It's an amazing feeling and the more you do it, the better it gets. The skin is a very sensitive organ and whether it's our own caress or another's, if we stroke our skin tenderly and with full attention it stimulates the flow of oxytocin, the feel-good bonding hormone that we get from a hug or after an orgasm.

If this exercise is too hard for you to begin with, start with the part of your body that you feel kindest towards and each day add another part until over time you are able to be kind and accepting towards your whole body.

EXERCISE 11: CONNECT TO SOURCE

Using my suggestions earlier in this chapter, do something three times in the next week that allows you to connect with the spaciousness of your inner source. You might want to experiment with a few different techniques. The clue is in the word 'spaciousness' – it's the best way I can describe the way my heart opens and the sensation of boundlessness that opens up in my mind when I connect to source. This does not necessarily have to be articulated or classified as a 'spiritual' experience, it's just that I don't know of any widely-enough disseminated vocabulary other the spiritual to describe it yet.

REFLECTIONS ON THIS CHAPTER

In this chapter we've been looking at how the process of change we're going through brings into focus all our relationships – with our bodies, with our deepest self and with others.

How has it been for you to start thinking about these things? Have you perhaps realised that you've been incredibly hard on yourself up until now and that maybe it's time you cut yourself some slack? Or maybe you've had some fresh thoughts about how others relate (or fail to relate) to you?

If you managed to do the 'Saying Thank You' exercise I hope you found it a simple but moving way of making a move back towards asking your body's forgiveness after years of treating it with disdain or abuse. It may have brought up some strong feelings of sadness or shame, which is to be expected. See if you can do the exercise regularly, and notice how each time you do it, your feelings shift a little… You might also want to check out some of my additional recommended reading on the subject, particularly the work of Brené Brown (see Appendix).

Sometimes, the very idea of connecting back to source can be incredibly provocative. The depth of betrayal by life some of us feel may also include a feeling of being betrayed by our beliefs. When bad things happen to good people and we are brought face-to-face with our powerlessness as human beings, such things can shake us to the core. Whatever your beliefs, a crisis of faith is a profoundly destabilising experience.

Choosing to re-engage with thoughts like this after such a crisis can be very challenging. How was it for you to start exploring these issues, and how do you feel about the idea of reconnecting to source? Did you attempt the 'Connect to Source' exercise and how was that for you? Or did you dismiss it as more ridiculous new-age nonsense? Please remember that 'source' does not have to be explored or experienced in a religious or spiritual context if that's not your thing. Find a way of relating to it that works for you – such as 'life force' or 'universal intelligence' for example – and connect to it however feels right to you.

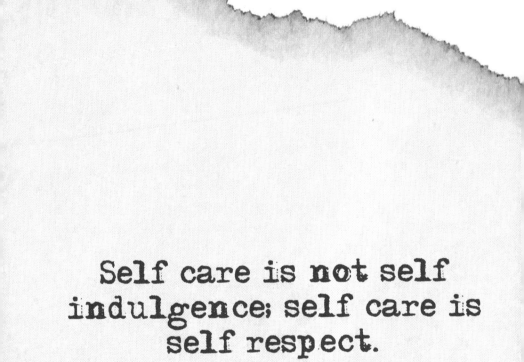

Self care is **not** self
indulgence; self care is
self respect.

CHAPTER 9

THE MOTHER WITHIN

THE GOOD MOTHER ARCHETYPE

Over the course of our time wanting to be mothers – for some of us from when we were young girls – we have dreamt about being mothers ourselves.

We've imagined what kind of mothers we would be, how we would do things differently (or the same), what we would name our children, how we would treat them.

We see our friends, family and complete strangers parenting their children and think, 'I wouldn't do it like that', or 'That's amazing, I'll remember that'. With our nephews, nieces, godchildren and the other children in our life we find ourselves drawing on a deep reservoir of instinct and learned behaviour as we relate to them, nurture them, teach them, comfort them and keep them safe.

> There is a part of us that is a mother even though we don't have a child of our own.

In our culture there are often examples of women who are biologically able to give birth but for whom being a parent is psychologically a major challenge. We are their opposite – women who are mothers in spirit, not in reality.

We are childless mothers – not just childless women.

In Jungian psychology, an archetype is something that exists as a potential within a personality until activated by the right circumstances, influence or experience. Everyone therefore has a 'mother archetype' and, for those of us who have longed to be mothers, those years of longing may have activated that archetype, yet it has never had a chance to be fully expressed. This may contribute to the 'aching arms' some of us report – a very physically uncomfortable feeling that can be experienced when our desire to nurture has been thwarted. It is something that mothers who lose their children also report experiencing.

This nurturing part of us finds expression in our care towards our loved ones, in mentoring young people, with our pets, our nephews and nieces and the other children in our personal and professional lives. But we can only offer them our tenderness, we don't get to give birth to them and help them shape themselves to face the world.

Ironically, for those us who work in caring professions and with children, our own wounding has given us a capacity for empathy that is a balm to others. We are loyal friends, patient daughters, loving partners, sensitive stepmothers, understanding sisters, kind aunts, civilised and friendly exes.

We are good women to others. So why are we so often cruel to ourselves?

MEET YOUR INNER BITCH

It's a shocking truth that many of us deny ourselves the tenderness and empathy that we so willingly and generously extend towards others. We talk to ourselves and treat ourselves in ways that we would never dream of doing to anyone else.

It seems that for some of us, from the moment we get out of bed there's a toxic running commentary going on in our head. Tuning into it can be a pretty shocking revelation. For a moment, imagine you were to 'turn the speakers on' and start hearing your internal commentary out loud.

It might sound something like this:

You stupid cow… you never get anything right.

Who put you in charge, you idiot?!

You look like shit today.

Forget it, don't even bother, you'll screw it up.

Have an extra portion fat-arse, it's not like anyone gives a shit about what you look like.

Don't screw up! If you lose this job, you'll never get another one!

You forgot the keys again you stupid moron!

No wonder you never got married, who'd want you?!

No one likes you, you loser.

Born to fail.

It's astonishing he hasn't left you already!

What's the point of reading this book, of trying to change – you'll never do it.

If you actually, physically *can't* say this stuff out loud, you're not alone. Because it may be that you realise that 'you' would *never* talk like that to anyone. You're just 'not that kind of person'. So what the hell do you think talking to *yourself* like that is doing to you?!

Wherever your harsh internal voice comes from, and whether you call it your Inner Critic, your Inner Bitch, your Top Dog or just 'you', it's time to understand it a little better in order to form a new and kinder relationship with yourself.

Kristin Neff, in her book 'Self Compassion' explains that the part of the brain that lights up during self-criticism is the amygdala – the oldest part of the human brain and the one that we share with reptiles. It would therefore seem that self-criticism is activated as a response to a perceived threat, as it's triggered by the same part of the brain that makes you jump when you hear a loud noise, even before you've had a chance to work out whether it's anything to worry about or not. Neff goes on to formulate that self-criticism is therefore trying to help us, to protect us. These days, we don't have to worry about being eaten by predators, but we do have to 'fit in' and so this primitive 'fight-flight-freeze' response is now used by our modern human brain to deal with social and emotional risks to our status, acceptability and lovability. Unfortunately, it also turns out that as a behaviour modification, self-criticism is, to use the non-scientific term, lousy! Self-kindness, on the other hand, 'allows us to feel safe as we respond to painful experiences, so that we are no longer operating from a place of fear'.[52]

So you see, there's nothing inherently 'wrong' with your Inner Bitch – it has its uses. Its vocabulary and values are created from what you learned from your parents, teachers and primary caregivers. Freud called this part of us our 'superego' and it's a crucial part of what becomes our adult conscience – but it's a building block, not the whole show.

> Our Inner Bitch has evolved to keep us safe from harm – but it seems
> that for many of us she's become a form of self-harm.

John Gottman, the famous American marriage therapist, has shown through hundreds of hours of close video analysis that for every critical comment or piece of feedback a couple gives each other it needs to be balanced with five positive comments or the marriage is in trouble. This 5:1 ratio proved to be accurate in 94% of the marriages Gottman analysed.[53]

The same 5:1 ratio has also been shown to be one of the hallmarks of outstanding business teams, with 3:1 being the 'tipping point' between teams failing and beginning to thrive.[54]

Do you give yourself at least five pieces of positive feedback for each critical one? Or even 3:1? Or did a voice pipe up that told you that if you did that you'd be 'spoiling yourself' or 'going soft' or any of the other messages you may have picked up? We live in a very perfectionist and achievement-oriented culture right now and there's a prevailing idea that 'pushing yourself' is more productive than 'being kind to yourself'. Somewhere along the way, self-kindness has become associated with a form of weakness, when in fact it's a source of incredible inner strength and resilience. Does the Dalai Lama seem like a 'weak' man to you?

We all know how much a critical comment from someone we love and respect can hurt. So just imagine what criticising *ourselves* harshly and with the relentlessness that many of us have learned *has* done to us and *is* doing to us. It's an act of psychic self-abuse and a way of punishing ourselves for being human and imperfect. Just like everyone else.

For example, when you're tired and need to take a nap, what does your Inner Bitch say? Does she say, 'Sweetheart, you look a bit tired, why don't you take a nap?' or is it more like 'You look like shit, but don't even think about sloping off for a nap – you've got way too much to do.

You're just lazy. You shouldn't have stayed up so late last night. It's your own fault. Just get on with it and stop complaining.'

This kind of relentless internal abuse wears us down, turns us off and puts us into a kind of permanent low-level battle with ourselves. In the end, it may be easier to numb out and avoid our inner world altogether than deal with this kind of toxic barrage. Turn the TV up louder, have another snack, pour another drink, stay late at work or stay in bed.

But by tuning out of our inner world because of our Inner Bitch, we also deny ourselves access to joy, creativity, dreams, inspirations, passions and love. This may be a factor contributing to the 'emotional deadness' that so many of us experience and which we fear is how we're going to feel for the rest of our lives…

> In order to even feel worthy of a meaningful and fulfilling life again,
> you're going to have to make friends with your Inner Bitch.

I don't know about you but for me, not having the family I dreamed of somehow 'confirmed' that my Inner Bitch had been right all along; that there was something fundamentally 'wrong' with me that I couldn't even get this 'simple' thing right, that 'everyone else' seemed to manage, often even by accident! My Inner Bitch wore me into the ground and, fuelled by the dark depression of grief, nearly took me out of the running altogether. There were days when I seriously wondered if I wanted any more of life as it had become so very painful, dark and utterly joyless. My inner world, devoid of love, became a torment to me. I hid it well around others, but alone at home I felt I was being eaten alive by my thoughts, my judgements, my criticisms. Each day I would wake up and try to 'get it right', but the bar was always too high and I would 'fail' and feel worthless, often before I'd even finished breakfast owing to the fact that my food choices weren't up to scratch. It was just toast. Again.

Your Inner Bitch isn't daft or evil – there's often wisdom in your self-criticism too – but there's no wisdom in running yourself down and abusing yourself every moment you're awake. You wouldn't expect a dog to thrive in those circumstances, let along a human being, let alone a woman recovering from the grief of childlessness and doing her damnedest to build a new life from the wreckage of her dreams.

Would you have talked to your children like this? Didn't think so – but there's a child inside you, and she's hurting, really hurting from how you're treating her.

From now on, I want you to start noticing what your Inner Bitch is saying and begin to change the language you use to yourself. Think how you'd say it to a dear friend or a young child.

You won't become 'soft' (yes, I feared that too), although you may 'soften' a little into becoming a kinder, more understanding person towards yourself. Another technique that Kristen Neff recommends is to put your hand on your heart as you talk to yourself – a gesture of physical tenderness, even from yourself to yourself, activates the 'care-giving' response in your brain rather than the 'flight-fight-freeze' response. It sounds silly, but try it. Put your hand on your heart, or on your arm if you're in public, and say something soothing to yourself either out loud or in your mind like 'Sweetie, I know you're really worried about this, but we've got through this kind of thing before and it's going to be OK'.[55]

> Beating yourself up doesn't work, I can guarantee you;
> I did it for years and all I got were bruises.

Healthy self-critique and harsh destructive criticism are very different: one builds confidence and enables us to learn from our mistakes; the other trashes self-esteem and leads to entrenched, repetitive and dysfunctional patterns of maladaptive coping. It's important to learn the difference. For me, I needed to learn how to be kind, loving and accepting towards myself *before* I could 'hear' the difference. These days, I actively seek critique from people whose opinion I trust. I feel that even if I hear something I don't like, I'll be able to handle it and that it will be helpful. I'm also able to make a decision on how to react and act on such information, rather than making a snap judgement such as 'I'm wrong' (which I'd interpret as 'I'm a bad person) or 'They're wrong' (which I'd interpret as, 'They're trying to hurt me').

Depending on your personality and your childhood experiences with your early carers and teachers, you will have a different 'tone' of Inner Bitch and a different degree of tolerance to criticism. However, learning to be kinder to ourselves is something we can all do and if we want to move forward with our Plan B, it's essential. We need our Inner Bitch on our side by training her to become our Inner Mother – protecting, guiding, teaching, nurturing and gently pointing out areas for improvement rather than yelling at us from the moment we wake up that 'You're useless!'

LEARNING TO BE A GOOD ENOUGH MOTHER TO OURSELVES

The influential 20th century English psychoanalyst Donald Winnicott developed the concept of 'the good enough mother': one who was not perfect, but robust enough to allow her child the freedom to explore and a strong enough sense of safety and security to do so.[56]

For me, this idea of being 'good enough', rather than either perfect or terrible, has been hugely transformational. I used to be an 'all or nothing' person when it came to self-care and found it hard to know the difference between self-care and self-indulgence, or between discipline and neglect. I believe that I probably inherited some of my mother's anxiety around these issues, at her knee and by her example, as she probably did from her own mother.

During my 40s I've come a long way towards developing healthier ways of relating to my inner world with the help of some excellent therapists, by attending 12-Step groups and through my ongoing training towards becoming a psychotherapist. I have discovered that my capacity for articulating my vulnerability is highly valued by others, as it often encourages them to share their own most tender spots. My vulnerability and my willingness to talk about it turns out to be one of my greatest gifts, not a weakness at all. *Take that, Inner Bitch!*

Now, before you think 'But I don't have a decade to sort this out!' I'm not suggesting that you need to do what I've done to get to the place that I'm at. Because during this decade of inner work, I've come to realise that I unpacked and worked through many of the core issues that can distress childless women – and that I've developed tools to deal with them and a network of support to help you get through them. I wish Gateway Women had been around 11 years ago although, to be frank, I wasn't ready then – I was still hopeful, still in denial at 38. It saddens me now to think how *different* those first few post-divorce years could have been if I had accepted *then* that I would probably never have children. But I guess I needed to go through that to get to where I am today, so it feels worth it – and anyway, I'm through with *What ifs...*

The result of this work has enabled me to stop seeing myself as 'damaged goods', but rather as a tender-hearted human with the capacity to heal, given the right encouragement and support. Just like you; just like all of us.

> Being 'good enough' also means that we give up beating ourselves up when we get being 'good enough' wrong.

For example, I use food to comfort myself when I'm stressed, lonely, tired or upset. I've done it since I was a child – wolfing down whole packets of sweeties in secret. It didn't show up in my weight for years – I was a skinny kid and teenager. As an adult, I gave myself an incredibly hard time about this and went on all manner of diets, gave up food groups and suffered from both under-eating and overeating problems. And I got plenty of support from the media for making my body the site of all my problems. I came to see myself as someone who 'had issues with food'. The thing is, I don't any more; it's a victim identity and I don't feel like one of life's victims anymore. Instead, I'm aware that food is something that can comfort me and that, within 'good enough' limits, it's not only absolutely fine, it's self care! I know what my 'good enough' limits are and I stick to them in a 'good enough' way – I don't keep sugary snacks in the house (biscuits 'talk' to me!) but if I feel like some chocolate I'll buy some and eat it. I've learned to read a desire for something sugary as a desire for some nurturing – so I've also learned to spend some time working out what it is that's creating that need: am I tired? Unwell? Overwhelmed? Lonely?

These days I nap when I'm tired; stay in bed when I'm ill; cancel appointments if I'm overwhelmed; seek out company if I'm lonely.

Sometimes my Inner Bitch wins and I don't nurture myself and instead I get stuck in a self-punishing regime of *Don't stop, Don't rest, Don't be ill, Don't need anyone.* The fact is, I don't get it right all the time and sometimes I have to fight through a wall of resistance in order to nurture myself. Dealing with being both single and childless along with working from home can sometimes mean that I'm on my own too much – which I have to keep a loving eye on as social isolation is fertile ground for my Inner Bitch.

But it's improving, I'm improving. And I've got 'good enough' at it to make a *huge* difference in my daily life. Each time I substitute a nurturing Inner Mother message for that of my Inner Bitch and discover that, after I've taken the nap, cancelled the appointment, turned down the offer or phoned a friend, that the world is still turning – it gets easier the next time. It's a little bit more data that proves that my Inner Bitch isn't always right. She's entitled to her opinion, after all, she's only trying to look out for me – but it's just an opinion, and a very 'young' one at that.

By taking action like this I am becoming the sort of 'good enough' Inner Mother to myself that I would have been to my own child or to the little 'Russian doll Jody' who lives within me: indulgent (within sensible limits), kind, honest and supportive. And not afraid to point out, with great love, where I might be going wrong sometimes.

Winnicott's work showed that the 'good enough mother' was actually *better* than the 'perfect mother': because a perfect mother (if she existed) would actually stifle our development. For us, being a 'good enough' version of ourselves is all that we need expect of ourselves. Perfectionism is another face of 'not good enough' and another classic platform for the Inner Bitch – a desperate way to maintain an illusion of control in an uncontrollable world.

> Give yourself a break. Try showing yourself some kindness and compassion instead of being harsh and judgemental. You'll see that the world doesn't actually fall apart.

It's an illusion that being mean to yourself is the only thing that keeps you 'in check'. You wouldn't expect a child or a puppy to do well with that kind of training, so maybe it's time to take a new approach with your relationship to yourself.

NURTURING THE MOTHER WITHIN

For those of us who wanted to be mothers but for whom it didn't work out, it's important to recognise that our desire to give, to nurture, needs an outlet in our lives.

If we *don't* have an outlet for that feeling, it may become 'stuck energy' and may even be what fuels some of the psychodramas we have going on with our Inner Bitch.

It can be hard to know what to do with our nurturing drive, particularly if we don't have a partner at this point and so are also starved of touch and intimate connection. Many of us have pets and this helps a lot, but then some of us deny ourselves that pleasure for fear of becoming the stereotypical childless woman with a cat or dog, whilst others are unable to have a pet for any number of reasons, even though they long to. And then some of us really aren't fussed about pets!

However, pets, partners or not, there is someone we *can* nurture and she's probably in desperate need of it – and that's ourselves. *Oh yes, I felt you pull back from the page then! Stay with me...*

It can feel hard even *contemplating* the idea of nurturing ourselves these days as it requires developing an intimacy with ourselves that we may have shut off from. We may also have to battle through ideas of 'self-indulgence' and 'self-obsession' before we'll even consider it.

However, for a moment, imagine you were a mother taking care of your child – would that have felt self-indulgent or would it have been loving and thoughtful?

What is Self Care?
Self care is *not* self-obsession.
Self care is *not* selfishness.
Self care is *not* self-indulgence.
Self care is self-respect.

EXERCISE 12: THE FEEL GOOD MENU

Choose an item from each of the 'courses' on the Feel Good Menu that follows and commit to doing one each day for the next week.

Some tips:

- Commit to doing one self-care action a day, or a couple per week – whatever you feel you can manage for now. It's important not to set yourself up to fail.

- If there is a 'course' that strikes you as totally nuts or particularly self-indulgent, that may indicate that this is an area of self-care that you've neglected for some time.

- If one of the suggestions *really* turns you off, that's probably an activity to choose rather than avoid!

- If there is any terminology in the Feel Good Menu that bugs you, change it to something that doesn't. Don't let that be the reason you skip this exercise…

- Some of these menu items could be listed under a different 'course' – after all, we're complex human beings, not a menu! Don't let your analytical mind get bogged down in the details, that's just a way of resisting doing it.

- Feel free to order off-menu! See the menu items as invitations and ideas to guide you rather than as absolute prescriptions.

- Stick the Feel Good Menu somewhere where you'll see it regularly. You'll find a version of it on the Gateway Women website if you want to customise it and print it out.

- Expect a surprisingly *huge* amount of internal resistance to doing this exercise, but do it anyway.

THE FEEL GOOD MENU

Warning: may cause happiness and peace of mind.

See appendix for further resources

Heart Course

Hug someone and/or ask for a hug.

Share how you feel with a trusted, loving non-judgemental friend – and ask them to refrain from giving advice unless asked.

Be vulnerable – it encourages others to be vulnerable with you – and creates a healing intimacy. Choose wisely...

Sing on your own or find somewhere private and yell at the top of your voice. I find this is wonderful for releasing anger, particularly if I do it in the middle of a field or somewhere I know no one will hear!

Choose to trust yourself. If in doubt, look in the mirror and ask your own advice.

Play with your pet, and if you don't have a pet, borrow someone else's.

Watch silly clips of cats on YouTube or anything that makes you laugh.

Call a friend or relative that you care about but haven't spoken to for far too long.

Watch a film that makes you laugh and/or cry and really let rip!

Spend time with someone in your life who nurtures you.

Head Course

Talk to yourself as you would talk to a dear friend or small child. Give your Inner Bitch a day off.

Stop reading women's magazines and practise going a whole day without beating yourself up about the way you look.

Keep a journal or start doing Julia Cameron's 'morning pages' to clean out the mental garbage.[57]

Say 'thank you' out loud to each part of your body as you bathe, shower or moisturise.

Take a deep breath and remind yourself that, 'This too shall pass'.

Write a letter to your younger self or your older self.

Make a list of your accomplishments, skills & qualities.

Go on a 'news fast' for a day, a week and then try for longer.

Make a list of 10 things to be grateful for every night before bed for a week.

Clean out your email inbox and unsubscribe from all newsletters etc. that you don't read. Take a break from Facebook and other social media sites.

Body Course

Take a nap without setting an alarm clock.

Cook yourself a healthy and delicious meal and set the table for yourself as an honoured guest.

Soak in a hot bath with wine, candles, music and a trashy novel. Give yourself permission to switch off. Don't take the phone into the bathroom!

Buy yourself some new underwear and get rid of all the 'tired' stuff.

Dance around the living room alone to your favourite music.

Give yourself a pedicure and paint your toenails a wild colour.

Go swimming, walking or cycling outdoors for at least 15 minutes. Or just sit with your face in the sun...

Walk barefoot on the ground for at least 15 minutes.

Do some gardening and weeding or tend to your houseplants.

Declutter your wardrobe and give away all the clothes you don't wear. Think, 'If this fitted me, would I wear it this season?' If not, let it go.

Source Course

Spend some time alone in nature and leave your phone at home.

Learn to meditate by taking lessons or listening to different guided meditation recordings– explore different tools and techniques until you find the one that's for you.

Choose a pack of goddess, angel or archetype cards and pick one every morning as 'guidance' for your day. This isn't magic – it's just a way of focusing your thought and intention for the day.

Pray in your own way each morning. Say 'thank you' more often than please – gratitude and joy are proven to light up the same areas of the brain.

Think of someone who may be lonely and give them a call.

Plan your funeral arrangements and create a beautiful way for your guests to celebrate your life. Write or update your will. Thinking about death is very life affirming.

Find a way to do a secret good turn for another person every day for a week.

Listen to a guided visualisation tape or recorded birdsong.

Forgive yourself for your mistakes. Forgive others theirs too.

Visit a sacred place. Whatever that means to you.

Reflections on this Chapter

In this chapter we've begun to explore some of our inner worlds – both our 'Inner Mother' and her shadow, our 'Inner Bitch'. We are all made up of shades of light and dark and indeed, one cannot exist without the other – but for many of us, finding out that we're not the only one that's staging a one-woman campaign against our self-esteem can be a huge relief! It can also come as quite a shock that a 'nice person' like us can be such a complete bitch inside our own heads…

How has it been for you to look at your inner world in this way? Did you manage to catch your Inner Bitch in the act of destructive criticism and did you practice shifting your language to something more self-compassionate and constructive?

For many of us, tuning into our harsh inner voice can be extremely illuminating because, perhaps for the first time in years, we realise that we have more control over how we feel than we realise. We've been bullying ourselves and the results have been predictably unhappy. Knowing that we can stop doing this can be a ray of hope that we're not doomed to feel awful about ourselves forever.

Did you commit to doing something from each course of the 'Feel Good Menu' and were you able to carry them out? Sometimes, the resistance we feel to doing something differently, even something that we think we're going to enjoy, can be really hard. It may also bring up some grief and sadness and therefore feel easier to 'put it off' for another day. Whether you did or didn't follow through with your intention, you may still have found it hard – either to realise how long it is since you've focused on doing something that made you feel good – or sad that the prospect of doing so turned out to be much scarier and more emotionally upsetting than you might have predicted. Remember, all change is destabilising to the ego, even the good stuff – so don't give yourself a hard time about it but choose to show yourself some self-kindness and self-compassion instead.

The 'Feel Good Menu' is not a one-week exercise – it's a lifelong one. Is it worth it? Well, when the prize is getting our mojo back, it definitely is! You've got nothing to lose but your unhappiness, and you can have that back anytime, free of charge.

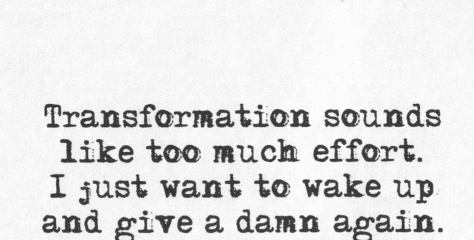

Transformation sounds
like too much effort.
I just want to wake up
and give a damn again.

CHAPTER 10

CREATING A LIFE FOR YOURSELF AS A CHILDLESS WOMAN

WHY IS CREATIVITY SUCH A SCARY WORD? (TERRIFYING, ACTUALLY!)

Creativity is one of those words that gets a reaction faster than almost any other word I know. It makes women in my workshops or groups take a sharp breath in and move backwards in their seats! Creativity seems to be one of the best words for making our Inner Bitch jump to attention and say, 'No thank you, we don't do *that* around here!' before you've even had a chance to open your mouth.

I've come to believe that creativity is one of the roots of recovery from involuntary childlessness. *Stay with me...* And that our instant discomfort with the very *notion* of creativity is actually a sign that we're on the right track...

The thing is, we may have become so comfortable with our 'Poor me, I couldn't have children' identity that we're actually a bit reluctant to let go of it. Paradoxically, your discomfort has become a place of safety because you're so used to it.

Our ego's job is to keep us safe in an unsafe world and it
does a great job of it by making *all* change seem like a threat.
And that includes creativity.

I mean, if we weren't so busy feeling sorry for ourselves and blaming
how unimpressed we are with our lives on our childlessness, we might
actually have to *do* something about it – and that 'doing something
about it' involves change. For those of us who have suffered so much
from our dream of motherhood not coming true, dreaming a new dream
takes courage. Huge courage with big boots on!

I have a theory (road-tested to exhaustion in my own life) that we
only change when the pain of changing becomes less painful than the
pain of not changing. And so I can be as stubborn as a mule when it
comes to hanging onto things that make me miserable because they feel
'familiar'. Call me a martyr, call me a masochist or just call me human.
I've come to understand that change (even good change) involves loss,
something that has to be let go of, and that because we've experienced so
much loss, we've become almost allergic to it.

Creativity and change are two aspects of the same thing; it's about
making something new happen. Bringing into being something that
would never have existed had you not been alive. But it brings a side
order of loss with it too.

One of the reasons creativity is so scary is that once we take that first
step we don't know where we're heading. We're building a new path to
a new destination in unknown territory and there's no guarantee that
when we get there we're going to like it. When you put it like that, it's
hardly surprising that many of us are too scared to take that first step.

But consider this. We've survived worse.

Although we may not know if we can handle anything else
'going wrong', deep down we know that as we've already survived the

unthinkable, how bad could it be, really? When I broke up from my first serious post-divorce romance I felt really low. But then I thought to myself, *If I can survive getting divorced from the love of my life I can survive this… I'll be OK. This too shall pass.* (An example of my Inner Mother giving me some kind and pragmatic support there.) I'm not asking you to become stoically immune to pain but instead to recognise that you can be vulnerable, nervous *and* incredibly resilient, all at the same time.

Sometimes, it seems outrageously unfair that not only did we not get to be mothers but that now we *also* have to take responsibility for our own happiness as well. Some booby prize, huh? But life's not fair – we've learned that. Letting go of that sense of entitlement is one of the keys to freeing us up to create our future.

FED UP OF CHANGE

Sometimes when I'm feeling fed up of transformation and the pain of letting go, I get a bit nostalgic for denial. For those days when motherhood was a 'when'…

I think one of the things that makes us fear change is the idea that 'letting go' of the past means 'losing it forever' but that's not been my experience.

Since that moment on a Tuesday afternoon in 2008 when I realised that I would definitely *never* be a mother, I've been in a spin cycle of change. But those changes have not erased my past. Rather, who I was when I wanted to be a mother has integrated with the person I've become, and keep becoming. I have *expanded* my idea of who I am and that includes *who I was then*. This expansion of my identity has also given me the necessary perspective to be much kinder to the person I was back then. And in turn, that's enabled me to forgive myself for some of the dumb decisions I made, and often blamed others for. I've downgraded my resentment against the world, myself and other people and that's made my reality a lot easier to inhabit.

These days change, creativity and letting go are my constant companions. And we bitch at each other from time to time, like all constant companions tend to do.

Giving Birth is Not the Only Act of Creation

If you accept my definition of creativity as the power to make something exist in the world that wouldn't have existed unless you'd been alive, giving birth to another human being can be seen as the primordial creative act. It's also a creation that keeps evolving and growing and changing.

For millennia, men have both feared and revered women for their power to bring forth life. The entire structure of patriarchy (literally 'rule of the father') is about putting some kind of boundary around a woman's fertility to ensure that her children are definitely that of the *known* father and therefore able to inherit *his* property.

> Giving birth isn't the *only* creative act. Neither is it the only profoundly energising and meaningful one.

It's important for us as childless women that we find *another* way to create – to leave our stamp upon this earth and give birth to something that wouldn't have existed had we not been alive.

Shadow Artists

Julia Cameron, in her influential book about rediscovering our creativity 'The Artist's Way'[58] writes of the 'shadow artist'. This is someone who longs to express themselves creatively but feels too hemmed in by their fear to do so. So, instead of singing, for example, they work for an opera company; instead of acting, they become an agent; instead of becoming an inspiring public speaker they work as an event organiser. It's as if they want their dreams to keep them warm, but they don't want to get burnt. But by getting close, but not quite close enough, after a while they feel frustrated and locked-out. Often they then burn out.

For those of us who wanted to be mothers and who live in a world full of other people's children, and maybe even work with them, we too need to be aware of this. We're not going to get to be a mother by the back door and, much as it's (sometimes) wonderful to be around children, in forcing ourselves to do so just to prove that 'we're OK' with not having our own we may be doing ourselves a real disservice.

As we get the support we need to do our grief work we will notice that our desire and reactions to being around children change. I went through a stage of finding them adorable, then annoying, then heartbreaking and then I became quite bored of them. These days, it depends on the individual child because I now relate to them as *individuals* rather than as living examples of what I don't have. I'm also OK with feeling annoyed if my peace gets wrecked in an adult-orientated public place like a restaurant. I no longer translate that into *I would have been a terrible mother and that's why it didn't happen.* I just allow myself to feel a bit annoyed whilst also feeling compassion for the parents who are usually all-too-aware that their child is being a bit of a pain. And if they're not aware, I might even be brave enough to be the one adult in the room that gently points it out to them.

> We may not feel nourished by being around children until we have found a way to nourish ourselves.

Until we find that thing that makes our soul sing again, being around children may be a bittersweet experience. But once we've found it we'll be able to connect with them from an authentic place, and they'll feel that too.

I remember when I was about seven or eight and an uncle and aunt of mine came to visit. They always used to bring me such lovely presents, much more thoughtful ones than I was used to getting. However, I also remember that they used to make me nervous – they paid me a level of attention I simply wasn't accustomed to – 'Go outside and play' was what most adults said to me if I wanted to talk or listen to them. It wasn't until I was a grown up childless woman myself that I understood that the nervous feeling I had felt around them was because they were an involuntarily childless couple. I felt their 'difference' and it bothered me. As a young bride, I asked this uncle to give me away in church in place of my father (whom I have never met), not knowing that as I did so that I too was destined for a life excluded from the rituals of parenthood.

These days, I'm mostly fine with the fact that I don't have children. Some days are easier than others, but occasionally I wonder if I miss the identity and camaraderie of motherhood as much, or more, than having a child in my life. For decades I took for granted the company of my female peers – through schooldays, adolescence, young womanhood and going through my 20s and 30s. And then, over time, as all of them moved to this new place called 'motherhood', I gradually realised that I was increasingly alone – and just at the time when it felt like I needed my friends the most. I thought it was just me, but it turns out that this is an experience many of us have to deal with. It is a cruel irony that childlessness can also involve the loss of our peer group, as well as the loss of our future family. We are exiled from both our past life *and* our future life. What our girlfriends, now busy round-the-clock with motherhood, often fail to realise is that it's rarely just they that are 'too busy' to stay in touch with us – it's most, or sometimes all of our 'old' friends. It can be very painful for us to see them moving on to new friendships, going on holiday and away for weekends with other families, whilst we struggle to get a date in our diary with them months ahead only to have them cancel at the last minute. After a while, we stop bothering and wonder if they'll notice. They rarely do.

Being single and childless as I am at the moment sometimes feels like I drew life's ultimate short straw, so much that we refer to it as 'double-whammy' in the Gateway Women online community – but then I look at some other couples' relationships and I'm reminded that I don't fancy a picnic on the grass over there! And to a great extent it's been my *choice* to be single – I needed to let this enormous transformation from being 'still hopeful' to being 'childless' settle in. It's changed me so much and I needed to work out who I was and what I wanted from a relationship if it's not about creating a family. And what I have to offer too, because I'm simply not interested in being a partner/wife in the way I understood before. No way.

> Increasingly, my life feels like a blessing just the way it is. And I simply cannot believe that I'm able to write that, let alone genuinely feel it.

CHILDFREE ARTISTS

Perhaps one of the reasons that there are so many more famous male artists than female ones (after deducting socio-economic-cultural factors) may be partly because men are drawn to art as a way of gaining access to the sacred realm of creativity that is contained in the miracle of birth.

Perhaps because men *can't* give birth, instead they choose to dance it onto canvas, breathe it into marble or conjure it from the air and into music...

Some of the world's most well-known female artists are childless or childfree – Frida Kahlo and Georgia O'Keefe are two examples that spring to mind – and the single-minded focus of the dedicated artist is not an easy one to combine with hands-on motherhood. As the English writer Cyril Connolly wrote: 'There is no more sombre enemy of good art than the pram in the hall'[59] and Virginia Woolf, though she longed for children in her marriage, also knew that the role of the 'Angel in the House'[60] (what has now been rebranded the 'domestic goddess') was an all-consuming one that left no room for the identity of the artist.

Having spoken to contemporary female artists who are childfree-by-choice, they don't feel that they're missing out on something essential because their work fulfils that space in them. They have chosen to put their creative life force into their art, and it shows in their work.

That's not to say that it isn't possible to be *both* a mother and an artist. Indeed, one of my favourite contemporary British artists, Jenny Saville, has been further inspired by motherhood and also by her children's creativity: 'the total freedom they have, scribbling across paper, the way they paint without any need for form. I thought: I fancy a bit of that myself.'[61]

The Playful Child Within

Like Jenny Saville watching her children play, it's quite easy to observe that creativity and play are one and the same thing. Through play, through creativity, children shape their understanding of the world.

The unmanifest interior world of their imagination interacts with the manifest exterior world of observable reality and in these interactions they form their own concepts of how life and reality operate. They are creating the world in their own image, brick by brick, drawing by drawing, game by game. Play *is* work for children. It's not something they do 'for fun'. It's life itself being brought into being.

Although if asked, most people would say that the opposite of play is 'work', the play researcher Dr Stuart Brown has said that, 'The opposite of play is not work. The opposite of play is depression.'[62]

The lack of joy, movement and playfulness that so many of us childless women experience as we come to terms with the heavy reality of not having children may possibly be because we are partially stuck in the depression phase of the grief cycle. Anhedonia, the inability to feel pleasure, is a symptom of depression.

For me, it seemed an added grief to bear that the things that used to bring me pleasure no longer seemed to have any effect on me. I'd go for a walk in the park to kick through autumn leaves and feel stupid and retreat to the café; I'd go swimming, only to find the noise of the public baths deafening and the whole experience damp, cold and unsatisfying. My bicycle stood chained to the railings with flat tyres for years because the pleasure of cycling through London streets and feeling the air on my face had vanished. Those years felt like a kind of death-in-life to me. Not knowing that I was grieving the family I never had, I thought this was just what middle-age felt like and some days I really wondered if I could face an entire life that felt this zombie-like.

In the Gateway Women groups and workshops, I often see a similar-looking face staring back at me as I met in the mirror every morning for about three years. And when I suggest the idea of play or creativity, of doing something spontaneous, they look panicked.

> Stuck in grief, in sadness, we forget how to play.
> And in doing so we forget how to live.

We know it, we feel it, but we haven't got a clue what to do about it. Everything feels too hard. Or, we have the germ of an idea but are too scared to take the next step. It's as if life has turned mean on us and we don't know if we can face any more disappointments when this one, not having children, feels like it's nearly wiped us out.

ILLNESS AS A DEFENCE AGAINST CHANGE

When I talk of Plan B what I mean by that is shorthand for a 'life of meaning'. Plan B is a life that gets you out of bed in the morning and that you feel excited to talk about when someone asks you about your life.

Many of us have become defined by our failure to become mothers and the loss not only of our families, but also the camaraderie and belonging of motherhood. Of course, motherhood isn't always rosy and if we cast our minds back to our *own* childhoods we may recall the way that the identity of motherhood didn't always sit comfortably with our own mothers.

But losing out on that identity, especially if we've spent a huge chunk of our life so far hoping and trying to make it come true, can leave us hollowed out, formless and feeling almost invisible.

When we look at childfree-by-choice women (and there are all varieties of them, just as there are all varieties of us, and of mothers) we might envy them just a little. After all, they *knew* they didn't want to be mothers, lived in a time when it was possible to make that choice and got the life they wanted. They're not hollowed out husks, invisible, lacking identity. Neither are they all defined by their childfree status. By never making motherhood a goal, not becoming a mother hasn't defined them either. They are women, not childless women.

Losing the possibility of the mother identity can be so devastating to us that we may subconsciously want to hang on to it by remaining stuck in grief. And one way that this might show up as a way of resisting creative living is through illness.

Many of us talk of *my body* as if it were something separate from us; a fleshy, watery envelope that we inhabit and that does strange things that we don't always agree with. But this is a way of thinking that simultaneously separates us from our bodies whilst also allowing us to avoid taking responsibility for ourselves.

If there's something we don't want to deal with yet, like acknowledging that we need a new idea for our life now that we know we're not going to become mothers, a way of avoiding that can be to develop illnesses.

The word 'psychosomatic' is often bandied around like some kind of slightly distasteful neurotic habit, but with that word the medical profession acknowledges that the mind is capable of creating physical symptoms that are genuine – that an illness can be, in part, created by the mind. Another of my favourite expressions is the 'placebo effect' – in which the ability of the mind to heal the body *without* the intervention of drugs is both expected and allowed for during clinical drug trials.

So you see, you don't have to have a dream catcher on your porch to acknowledge that our minds and bodies work together in ways that are, as yet, little understood by modern medicine to create both illness and wellness.

Denial, the first stage of the grief process and often the first stage of the change process, is a ripe ground for psychosomatic illness. Whilst I was in the depths of denial about my infertility and the car-crash my marriage had become I came down with every illness going around the office, as well as food poisoning, migraines, tooth abscesses and a binge-eating disorder that culminated in me sleepwalking and eating at night.

I spent the best part of a year too ill to think. Which was exactly what I wanted. I didn't *want* to think. I wasn't ready.

If you are unable to contemplate your Plan B because of an illness, or a series of minor illnesses, it might be worth listening to your body, because it's *definitely* listening to you. It might be that you are forcing yourself to take the next step before you are ready and that what you really need right now is some support in order to process your grief. Or it might just be that you're scared of change and being ill gives you a type of solid identity that you're not ready to give up yet. You may also be burnt-out and in need of a period of profound rest. Once upon a time, we used to have a thing called 'convalescence'. Our need for it at a physical level still exists, it's just that our culture doesn't have space for it. We're all meant to be busy 'doing' something – all the time. Sometimes, it seems that the only way to get that kind of rest is to burn out so that we have no other option. It's happened to me a few times and I'm now much more alert to the warning signs and let my Inner Mother take charge at that point and not my Inner Bitch!

It's important that you don't think I'm saying that all illness is in your mind and that therefore it's *all your fault*. I am not a medical expert and I'm only drawing from my own and others' experiences that I know of. Many of us are childless because of chronic conditions and I'm not saying that positive thinking or any such *woo-woo* is going to make ME, CFS or any of the other conditions that stop us in our tracks go away. There is a plague of positive thinking that has come over from the US (and which perhaps reaches its most toxic levels in the vernacular of cancer and infertility treatments) that can be oppressive and shaming – *I had a negative thought about my treatment/recovery chances and that's why it's not working.* Barbara Ehrenreich, the American feminist and social journalist, wrote an excellent book about this called 'Smile or Die: How Positive Thinking Fooled America and the World' having been exposed to the tyranny of such thinking during her own cancer treatment.[63]

So, if you have a chronic illness, please don't add this to your list of things to blame yourself for – it's not going to help. However, if you are ill because you need time to cocoon and this is the only way you know how to give yourself permission to do so, then this is where you need to be. But if you know, deep down, that your cocooning time has passed and that you're stringing it out because you're terrified of taking charge of your life again, then maybe it's time to take a risk with a tiny bit of creativity and see what happens.

You know the answer: trust yourself. And if you're not sure, experiment. Do the exercise at the end of this chapter in the smallest way you can and see how it makes you feel. Listen to that. Sometimes not becoming a mother can leave us with a profound sense of mistrust in ourselves, so it's hardly surprising that we find it hard to initiate change.

> Learning to trust your ability to know what's best for you can be as healing as actually *doing* what's best for you.

Your relationship with yourself has taken a hell of a battering and there's no shame if you need time to rebuild. After all, blowing up bridges is a lot faster than building them.

WARNING! 'THERE BE DRAGONS'

I believe that reconnecting with our creativity and debugging whatever terrors the word brings up for us is an absolutely vital part of not only recovering from our childlessness, but also in creating a life that works for us. And that's what Plan B is all about: creating a new life for ourselves that has meaning, passion and purpose at its core.

What that means for each of us is different. We need to have a conversation with our soul and slay a few dragons too. We need to get off the sidelines of our life, and become our own heroine again.

In the next chapter we're going to start constructing your first Plan B. It will probably be the first of many because as you grow, heal and change, your needs and desires will change too. We are always work in progress just like everything else on earth.

However, with our tendency to be harsh and exacting with ourselves, we may make our first Plan B all work and no play. And that's not going to get you out of bed in the morning, is it? So, this week's exercise is to help awaken your playful side again. *Yes, I heard you groaning at the back!*

EXERCISE 13: GETTING CREATIVE TO FIND YOUR PLAN B

Grab a pile of Post-It notes. Write each word or phrase that comes to mind in response to this exercise on a separate Post-It note (or separate small pieces of paper).

Answer the prompts below with single words or short phrases and write each one separately.

1. Write down the answers to the following questions. Do it spontaneously and write down your first thoughts. If nothing comes to mind, move onto the next prompt. Try not to think about it too much, or what your answers might 'mean':

- What five words or phrases pop up when you think of the word 'creativity'?

- What five things or games did you love doing or playing when you were a child?

- What do you wish you hadn't 'given up' from when you were a child?

- What adult activity puts you into a place of 'flow' (where time seems to soften and you are completely absorbed and at peace)?

2. Now, spread out all your answers (if they are on Post-It notes, stick them on a wall or window). Jumble them all up. Can you see any patterns or themes emerging? Group them accordingly.

Choose a 'baby step' that you can commit to this week to bring one of these themes alive. It doesn't have to be a huge commitment (that's your Inner Bitch talking) and it definitely mustn't be worthy or productive. In fact, the smallest, least complex and more frivolous the better!

Depending on your personality and abilities what's fun for you might be hell for someone else, so please don't feel constrained by the following random examples:

- Listen to music that you love and haven't listened to in a while.

- Go to the kind of place 'you used to love' such as an art gallery, craft centre, museum, tool store, art shop, bookshop, farmers' market, garden centre, junk yard or library – anywhere that inspires or intrigues you but which you notice you've been avoiding recently. Buy a postcard or some small thing as a memento. Notice what you are drawn to.

- Spend time going through your clothes and wear something that makes you look and feel great – just for the hell of it.

- Declutter your bedroom, rearrange the furniture, give it a good clean and make it feel special again.

- Get your camera out and go for a walk. Photograph anything that catches your attention. Print out the pictures and stick them up or perhaps share them with others in the Gateway Women online community.

- Do some sewing or baking, purely for fun.

- Write a poem.

- Make a cushion or other craft project.

- Drive a new route to work, eat a different lunch, talk to different people.

- Read a biography of a childless woman you admire (If you need some inspiration, check out the Gateway Women Gallery of Childless & Childfree Role Models on Pinterest).

- Plant some new flowers in your garden, buy yourself fresh flowers, get creative with some flower arranging.

- Fix something that's broken with your own hands: the lawn-mower, the computer, the kitchen cupboard, your motorbike – whatever feels like the most fun.

- Go horse-riding, wild swimming, ice-skating, rock-climbing, salsa dancing or karaoke singing – whatever you either 'used' to do or always wished you 'could' do.

REFLECTIONS ON THIS CHAPTER

In this chapter we've been looking at how our childlessness and our creativity are linked, often in surprising ways. These kinds of new thoughts can often stir up a lot of old memories and perhaps some more grief. This is not a sign that you are weak or that you are not capable of healing and creativity – in fact it means exactly the opposite. A healthy psyche will not allow us to feel feelings that we are yet not capable of coping with; that's what denial is for. If you can feel it, you can heal it.

The notion that you may have developed illnesses as a defence against change can be quite provocative – did it give you pause for thought or did the very idea of it make you furious?! And how about the idea that birth is not the only creative act? Did it give you a surge of hope or perhaps you found it preposterous because the idea that anything could 'replace' motherhood is not something you're ready to give houseroom to yet?

It doesn't matter where you are in your responses to these ideas but only that you honour where you're at and start from there. Pretending, even to yourself, that you feel other than you do isn't going to move you forward. We've all spent more than enough time already pretending that we're more OK with our childlessness than we really are; we don't need to keep up that pretence in private or with other childless women.

And how did you respond to the idea that creativity and change are aspects of the same thing? Did it give you some insights into why creativity can feel a bit scary sometimes, or did it perhaps confirm your belief that creativity is just something for 'other people'?

Did you attempt the exercise or was the c-word too big for you to deal with? Sometimes, accessing our playful, creative nature can be quite hard to cope with because it may show us how far we've gone from that part of us. Conversely, it can feel so good that we feel guilty that we've denied it to ourselves for so long. Then again, it might be that creativity is already an integral part of our life, and so we may begin to wonder whether our passion and commitment to it is one of the reasons we ended up without children…

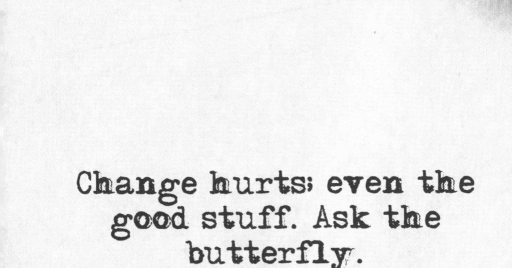

Change hurts; even the
good stuff. Ask the
butterfly.

CHAPTER II

PUTTING YOUR PLAN B TOGETHER

DIY Happiness

Because we don't have children we can't delegate the major part of our happiness, fulfilment and meaning to our role as mothers and our delight in our children – we have to do it for ourselves. And the feedback loop is invisible – no cheery little people smiling and hugging us, no knowing smiles of approval from other parents, no special day in the calendar to tell us how wonderful we are and how much we mean not just to our family, but to the whole world.

Whilst motherhood is a lifetime of hard work the results are tangible (even if you don't like them or they bring you great sadness) and once your child is born, usually irreversible. However, creating a life of meaning as a woman without children is a promise to ourselves that no one forces us to keep and which has to be renewed daily. No one's going to take you to court for neglecting *yourself*.

As a childless woman, no one's going to jump on your bed at 6am and remind you that you promised to:

- Write that book.
- Finish decorating your home so that you're not too embarrassed to invite people round.
- Change your job to one that doesn't make you spend more than you earn in therapy just to cope with it.
- Move to Paris; or get the hell out of Paris.
- Stop dressing like your house just burnt down.
- Meditate daily.
- Travel up the Amazon.
- Retrain as a garden designer.
- Volunteer at the animal refuge.
- Be kinder to yourself.
- Enter the world chess championships.
- Cook something that doesn't come in a packet.

It's all up to us. We are the grown-ups. We get to decide where we're going now. We're reluctant and accidental pioneers in raw new territory; there aren't any maps and precious few roads.

If you feel a little daunted and wonder whether you're up to the job, take heart. I think you'd have to be a risk-hungry adventurer not to feel a *bit* daunted and therefore more likely to be half-way to Alaska by now rather than reading this book. I don't know many women like that; you don't tend to meet them in bookshops.

I often wonder if one of the side effects of becoming a parent is that you realise (probably with a shock) that you are now *definitely* one of the grown-ups. For those of us who are childless we have to take that step alone, invisibly and, as usual, without anyone encouraging us or giving us a *woop-woop* when we do it. In fact our families, friends, society and employers often unconsciously treat us as if we were bizarrely-aged children compared to our sisters, colleagues and peers who have become mothers.

I don't know if you've ever been away from home for an extended period, living in another city perhaps or maybe even another country. The experience has changed you but when you get back, nothing seems to have changed and, after a few weeks, everyone forgets that you'd even been away. Being childless-by-circumstance and living your Plan B is a bit like that. No one's going to notice much or really be that interested, but we ourselves are changed profoundly, forever.

So, like I said, it's up to us... and we don't even *have* to do it. There is an alternative; we can always stay where we are for a bit longer, until we're ready. Or we can stay stuck for a lifetime, marinating in a sense of feeling hard done by that harms no one except us. Eventually that gets old. Or we do.

And the alternative? We can make the best of our lives anyway. No one but us can do it, and no one but us cares. It's not like anyone's ever going to accuse us of being a 'bad mother'. There are no gold stars in life for being a good childless woman, unless you become a saint. And it's worth remembering that mothers may well have to deal with this stuff later, once their children have left home. But they have a name for it: 'empty nest syndrome' and get sympathy, empathy, understanding and column inches to help them deal with it...

Debunking some Plan B Fairy Stories

'Plan B' is another way of saying 'creating a life of meaning' – it just sounds more pragmatic and do-able than a 'life of meaning'. A life of meaning sounds like a bit of a stretch right now, doesn't it?

If you think Plan B is a chance to change your career or get busy so that you don't feel so sad, you're only scratching the surface; this is a chance to create a life that makes you soar.

However, before you get too excited by the idea of 'soaring', a word of warning: a fantasy Plan B can be very seductive to us right now. It sounds like the pot of gold at the end of the rainbow; the place where everything is going to be OK, finally; our happy ending.

In the feedback forms filled in after Gateway Women groups and workshops there's often a request for 'more on Plan B please' and I've created a lot of material around it. But lately I've come to understand that I'm not really being asked for more material. In some cases the unspoken message is, *Can you please tell me how to sort my life out – I've tried and made a complete mess of it – you seem to have managed it – could you have a go with mine?*

And the answer is this: even if I could, it wouldn't work. It'd be as likely to work out as if I set you up on a blind date. Only you know your heart and soul's desire.

Because, you see, Plan B isn't an idea; it isn't even a plan when all's said and done: it's a process. A process of healing, of growth. And no one can do your healing for you; you can't outsource that.

SO WHAT IS A PLAN B?

- Creating your Plan B is about having the courage to take risks again when you feel that you've taken enough risks to last a lifetime, and *look* where it got you!

- Creating your Plan B is about learning to trust your instincts and follow your hunches again, despite what your Inner Bitch, your partner, your family, your friends, your boss and the wider world thinks.

- Creating your Plan B is about finding out who you are again once you drop the 'baby story' and having the faith that there *is* something left; a diamond to be found in the rubble.

- Creating your Plan B is about experimenting with your life and opening up that part of you that dares to dream again, when your last dream nearly killed you.

- Creating your Plan B is about having the self-belief that you deserve to have a happy and meaningful life despite the fact that society, your family and your peers have pretty much given up on you. You damn near gave up on yourself...

- Creating your Plan B means making changes to your relationship with yourself, the result of which will cause a ripple of change throughout all your relationships, whether you, or they, like it or not.

- Creating your Plan B means giving up some of the comfortable benefits of being one of life's 'victims' and starting to notice when you're making excuses for yourself.

- Creating your Plan B *also* means learning to be kinder to yourself as a way to encourage your growth and healing and to allow yourself to become the mother to yourself that you would have been to your children.

- Creating your Plan B means thinking about the future, about your old age, about what kind of footprint you want to leave in this world instead of the family you thought you'd have.

- Creating your Plan B is about taking responsibility for yourself and letting go of the idea that someone or something is going to save you. You don't need saving, sorry.

- Creating your Plan B is a radical, line in the sand way of saying to yourself: 'I matter'. Which in turn will start to show up all the things in your life that *aren't* working and which no longer serve you.

- Creating your Plan B is about creativity and change. About dignity and courage. About honouring yourself, standing up for yourself, valuing yourself. It's about paying attention to what matters to you, so that you can offer the best of yourself to your life, and to others.

- Creating your Plan B is about creating a life that fits you from the inside out and learning to accept that others may or may not get that, and that what they think is not actually all that important, frankly!

- Creating your Plan B is about creating a life that, when it's over, you think, 'Well, that was worth it!'

- Creating your Plan B is about...

> We each have the power, right now, to change our relationship to both our past *and* our future. It starts by giving ourselves permission to dream again.

So, if you think Plan B is something that's going to enable you to avoid pain and live an easy life, I'm afraid it's not going to happen. Because nobody gets to have a life like that and, even if you did, you'd be bored out of your mind.

Yes, we may look at other women and think, 'Well, her life's a complete picnic!' but we're wrong. *Nobody's* life is free of disappointment, suffering, disease, ageing, loneliness and death. The human condition affects us all. And that includes the desire to compare ourselves to others and feel hard done by.

WHAT ABOUT THE CATERPILLAR?

The metaphor of a caterpillar becoming a butterfly is often used when talking of transformational change and the story usually focuses on the moment that the butterfly emerges from the chrysalis: this beautiful, elegant creature born from a caterpillar.

> Change hurts, even the good stuff. Transformation doesn't feel like transformation – it feels like everything in life has gone to hell and nothing makes sense any more.

But this gets on my nerves. What about the caterpillar? How do you think the caterpillar felt when one day it found itself being entombed in a chrysalis and its entire body started turning to mush? To become a butterfly, the caterpillar has to completely dissolve, right down to the cellular level, and reform. I bet that hurts!

It's only afterwards, when we're out of the chrysalis, that we can look back and say: 'I'm really glad I'm not a caterpillar any more; that was worth it'. But until then, we have to have a lot of faith that at some point, things will make more sense.

When we were young women we knew that we'd have to 'make our life happen'. We probably spent much of our adolescence and teenage years mentally and emotionally preparing ourselves for adult life. We thought about how we'd shape the life we wanted and mostly, we felt up to the challenge. That part of us is still there – and she's smarter than she was when you were 20. She's probably also more fearful, but that's wisdom for you.

Whether you're ready to start making changes right now is something only you know. For me, I know that change is on the horizon when I feel utterly and completely frustrated with some aspect of my life and myself. I'm beside myself with confusion and I know that I simply *have* to do something about it or I feel I'm going to implode. But I often don't know what it is I have to do, although somehow I also *do*, I just don't want to admit that I know what it is! It's ugly and messy and often involves tears and a whinge or rant at one of my dear friends who insists on telling me that it's all going to be fine! I get migraines, back-ache, avoid phone calls and eat a lot of cookies. I overdramatically resign myself to being in a foul mood for the rest of my life!

And then, I realise that something's shifted... Whatever it was that was rumbling below the surface comes into view and is translated into a new thought, new energy, a new decision, a new behaviour, a new insight. My migraine passes, my backache eases and I start eating vegetables again. My good temper returns and I start picking up my voicemails.

Because I'm not naturally one of life's great risk-takers, I need to let my frustration (a form of anger) build up a head of steam in order to help me push through my resistance and let the shift happen. I rarely know what the shift *is* until it's underway. I'm *so* not psychic – I often don't even know what *I'm* thinking!

The good news is that I've noticed that this cycle is getting shorter with repetition. I suspect that one of the side effects of recovering from the grief of childlessness is that I trust myself more and that's making taking risks less risky. Because these days I trust that whatever happens, I'll cope. After what you've been through, couldn't you say the same? I mean really, how much have you coped with already?

> Your Plan B is not a contract with your future self to meet certain goals. It's not a vision board, a bucket list or some worthy resolution. It's a new way of living – one where you reach out for life rather than sit back and wait for it to disappoint you.

Your Plan B will change over time; it will evolve, as you do.

I never thought my Plan B would be to write this book and speak up for childless-by-circumstance women. I thought I was becoming a psychotherapist. Indeed, I still am becoming a psychotherapist (it's a long training!) but I am also becoming things that I don't even know about yet.

But most of all, I'm becoming authentically and unapologetically myself. These days I'm excited to see what I'm capable of and what the future brings, rather than feeling disappointed about what didn't happen.

And that's called having your mojo back.

FOLLOW YOUR BLISS

So, you get it: no one can tell you what shape your 'life of meaning' is going to have. It's a bit like falling in love – no one can tell you what it's like, only that once you've found it, you'll know.

If I can give you any clues at all, it would be this quote, from the famous mythologist Joseph Campbell: 'Follow Your Bliss.'[64]

I first came across this quote on a greeting card, the year before my marriage broke down. I bought the card to add to the pile I kept in my desk in readiness for other people's birthdays and special occasions, but I found that I could never bring myself to send it to anyone. Instead, I pinned it above my desk and it followed me around in the years following my divorce, always pinned where I was writing (or trying to write). It seemed to hold some essential truth that I was trying to grasp, but couldn't quite 'get'.

Looking back now, I realise that for a long time the reason I wasn't able to follow my bliss was because I didn't have any to follow. I was dead inside and it seemed that I'd felt that way for so long that I really didn't expect it to change. My life felt finished and I seriously wondered how I would find the energy to keep going for the rest of my life. I felt like the 'other' bunny in the Duracell bunny adverts, the one *without* the long-lasting batteries.

But the little Jody (aged about six) who lives as a Russian doll inside me – the one who used to write stories to read to the fairies in the woods; the one who lay on her back in cornfields and marvelled at the universe spinning around her – she was alive and well. She was the one who knew what that postcard meant and she was the one that hung onto it and kept pinning it above my desk. *She* knew what bliss was, which meant that somewhere I did too. I didn't need to learn it, rather I needed to *unlearn* a whole load of other crap that had got in the way.

The last time I remember seeing that card was around the time that I came out of denial about my childlessness and began thinking 'now what'? Some of my first Plan B ideas (although I didn't call it that then) were actually part of my grief work and weren't at all about bliss. For example, I seriously contemplated getting rid of all my possessions and moving to Laos to spend the rest of my life living and working in an orphanage on the Mekong river. (I blame the 'King and I'!) However, looking back on it now, I can see that parcelled-up in that plan was a mixture of romanticised tragic glamour, an escape from the reality of my pain and a desire to have my loss witnessed and understood by others through heroic self-sacrifice. I didn't think much about the orphans at all and it certainly wasn't about following my bliss – it was about following my pain.

Joseph Campbell said: 'If you follow your bliss, you put yourself on a kind of track that has been there all the while, waiting for you, and the life that you ought to be living is the one you are living.'[65]

The 6 Human Needs Model (Tony Robbins)

Before we move into creating your first Plan B, I'd like to introduce you to Tony Robbins' model 'The 6 Human Needs'.[66]

The 6 Human Needs are:

1. **Certainty** eg: predictability, security, safety, food, shelter, health, political stability.

2. **Uncertainty** eg: variety (because if nothing ever changed, you'd be bored!) This includes physical and mental stimulation, adventure, travel, surprise, change, risk, challenges, problems and opportunities. Good and bad.

3. **Significance** eg: feeling special and worthy of attention from others, having importance, status, feeling of value, creating a legacy, being of influence.

4. **Love & Connection** eg: relationships (including your relationship with yourself), friendships, family, faith, spirituality, community, nature, pets.

5. **Growth** eg: our response to change and adversity, character, depth, resilience, development, expansion.

6. **Contribution** eg: our legacy, our footprint, making a difference, standing up for what we believe in, moral courage.

These human needs are universal and, according to Robbins, a life well lived includes a balance of all of them. However, some of them overlap and perhaps even exclude each other at times, so it's more of a snapshot of a dynamic process than a static picture.

I first learned about the 6 Human Needs in a video of a TED talk called 'Tony Robbins Asks Why We Do What We Do.'[67] It's only 20 minutes long and it's worth watching, although you'll be glad that you've got my notes above to follow because wow, does he talk fast!

Robbins' model shares some similarities with other models, including Maslow's famous Hierarchy of Needs,[68] but what I like about the 6 Human Needs is that it can be used at both a micro and macro level as a snapshot of how our life is working for us at any time.

If you're averse to the idea that a model could be any help at all with understanding your life, these words from the mathematician George Box illuminate a great truth, namely that 'all models are wrong, but some are useful'.[69] A model is purely an intellectual way to simplify complexity so that we have an easier time extracting meaning from it. It's not 'the truth', just as a map is not the territory.

I like to represent Robbins' 6 Human Needs model as a circle divided into six segments, like a cake. That way, you can imagine each slice as one of the 6 Human Needs and consider how much of it you have in your life right now. The circle also gives the model the sense of a dynamic system of flowing and interconnecting needs, which feels more like life to me than a numbered list or the hierarchical, pyramidal structure of Maslow's model.

At different times in our life and at different stages of our development we tend to prioritise two of these Human Needs above others and this can become habitual. However, by doing so, we may be preventing ourselves from getting some of our other needs met. For example, if your way to feel 'significant' is to be the boss at home and at work, you may be feeling that you don't have enough 'love and connection' in your life, because your need to control others has pushed people away. Or, for example, if in your desire to 'make a contribution' you have locked yourself away from the world for a year to write a book, you may feel that your life has become a bit narrow and that your need for 'variety' or 'connection' with your friends and family has been neglected.

Preparation for Exercises 14, 15 & 16

It takes great courage to start dreaming again after all we've been through. It's quite likely that we've become overly serious about life and have lost contact, to some degree, with that playful part of us that used to daydream when we were young. Therefore, before we start our first Plan B exercise, we need to limber up a bit.

If, when you read through the following exercises, you think they're a bit trivial, I would invite you to slow down and do them anyway.

It's absolutely understandable that allowing yourself to dream again, to be playful again, to trust that despite your sadness life will turn out OK after all – is a lot to ask of yourself after what you've been through. But it's not going to magically 'go away' on its own.

> We don't get given a new life; we have to create it.

If you've been struggling with the grief of childlessness for years, you may find these exercises very hard, but I'd like to encourage you to have a go anyway. Sometimes, women in my groups and workshops find it really hard to write a single thing down, they find the instructions incomprehensible and the whole thing a bit of a mystery. If this is you, don't panic. What it *may* point to is that you're not quite ready to look into your future yet and that you might need to do some more grief work first. There's no shame in that, so please don't feel bad about it. Try to do the exercise anyway, and also commit to incorporating more grief work activities into your life. See Chapter 4 for more information and ideas.

Exercise 14: Time Travel

Grab a pile of Post-It notes. Write each word or phrase that comes to mind in response to this exercise on a separate Post-It note (or separate small pieces of paper).

Imagine you are 80 years' old and are looking back over your life. Allow yourself to daydream about the things that are going to happen between now and then *as well as* what has already happened. The only thing you cannot change in the future is that you cannot become a biological mother.

- **Achievements**: List the ten things that you are most proud of, including those things you hope or anticipate you *might* be proud of by the time you are 80.

- **Regrets**: Now, list the ten things you regret – those things you wish you'd done differently, or which you *anticipate* or *fear* you might regret by the time you are 80.

Arrange all your achievements and regrets into two separate columns. (Stick them on window or wall if possible). Stand back, and see if you can see any themes emerging.

Can you perhaps see how they map against the 6 Human Needs model? Are there perhaps a couple of Human Needs that you can see require your attention more than others?

You may see that some of your themes straddle more than one Human Need, for example:

- If one of your themes is something like 'doing well in my career', this might satisfy the need for Contribution as well as for Significance.
- Or 'Creating a beautiful home' might be part of your need for Certainty as well as for Growth.
- 'Travel' could be part of your need for Uncertainty as well as Contribution.

Only you will know what sense this makes to you, and what insights you gain from it. There are no right or wrong answers to this exercise – it's just a way to start loosening up what's important to you and getting some perspective on that.

So now we're going to let your Inner Bitch have her say on the matter...

EXERCISE 15: UNCOVERING YOUR RESISTANCE

Grab a pile of Post-It notes. Write each word or phrase that comes to mind in response to this exercise on a separate Post-It note (or separate small pieces of paper).

Try and write at least ten answers to each question below and don't be concerned if the same responses come up more than once...

Write down all your reasons, rationales, fears or negative thoughts about:

- Why you *haven't* done more of the things your older self is proud of.

- Why you *can't* do more of the things your older self wished you'd done more of.

- In a nutshell, what *has* stopped you in the past and what *will* stop you in the future?

When we do these exercises in the Gateway Women groups and workshops, most women find their list of 'achievements' as much fun as pulling teeth whilst their list of 'regrets' (even the ones that haven't happened yet) are much easier to identify. And as for the things that *have* and *will* get in their way – frankly it's hard to stop them writing!

The answers that they usually come up with are a variation on the following. Do yours fit under these same four categories?

1. Fear, including, amongst many varieties:

- Fear of rejection
- Fear of making a fool of myself
- Anxiety
- Scared
- Procrastination, indecisiveness
- Inertia, laziness
- Lack of discipline
- Fear of failure
- Fear of success

2. **Internal Resources** including:

- Low self-esteem
- Not smart enough
- Self-doubt
- Lack of self-belief, don't deserve it
- Lack of confidence
- Naturally inhibited
- Too shy
- Not listening to my instincts
- Jealousy, envy, inadequacy
- Depression
- Grief

3. **External Resources**

- Lack of knowledge
- Unlucky
- Poor health
- Too late
- Lack of opportunities
- Not enough money
- Not enough time
- Lack of talent
- Have to work too hard
- No energy left after work

4. Other People

- What others think
- My partner won't like it
- I'll get criticised
- Parental expectations
- Wanting to conform
- Living for others, not for me
- Being in the wrong relationship
- Listening to the wrong people
- Being let down or betrayed
- Poor parenting means I can't do it

When I ask everyone to put their Post-It notes up together on the wall and ask them to see if they can group them into categories (I don't tell them the 'titles' of the four categories beforehand), these four always show up. And the one with the longest list is always fear.

> Our Inner Bitch would have us believe that the reason we didn't get the life we wanted and *won't* get the life we want is because we're uniquely useless. *It's not true.*

These are women who have often never met before, all of different ages and from different backgrounds. Each of them sees, in front of their own eyes, that what they thought were *their own private weaknesses and failings are shared by everyone else in the room.*

What we're seeing here is universal. It's called the human condition. Different cultures may have slightly different versions of it, couched in slightly different language, but this stuff, what Steven Pressfield calls 'resistance',[70] is what *all* normal, well-adjusted individuals have to deal with.

Despite what we believe, we have not been *personally* singled out by fate to be fearful, worried about what others think, afraid to grasp new opportunities and unsure of our abilities to perform. It's normal.

Like everything else in the universe we are a combination of expansion and entropy; of growth and collapse; of forward and back; of love and fear.

Inside, we are all lovable and we are all scared. The trick is to know that everyone, no matter how successful or fearless they seem to you, feels the same.

It's time you gave yourself a break for being human. Because once you do, all the energy that went into telling yourself you're uniquely built to fail can go towards creating your Plan B instead.

BEWARE THE PRESSURE TO BE EXTRAORDINARY

I want to point out something very important about *who* and *what* your Plan B is for.

> Your Plan B is for *you*. It's about what a meaningful and fulfilling life would look and feel like to *you*. Not to anyone else.

There is a subtle pressure that because we are childless we have the space in our life to do something extraordinary. But the fact is, we don't have anything to 'make up for' because we haven't had children. That's just more shame talking – but it's a hard one to spot and an even harder one to resist sometimes. I call it the Mother Teresa complex.

It's very easy for us to fall into the trap of thinking that we should be 'doing' something with our life. Yet, if you had been a mother, would anyone (including you) have expected such things of you? Why should you have to be Mother Teresa just because you don't have children? And indeed, why shouldn't mothers be allowed big dreams and goals too?

This is another form of the 'not good enough' refrain of shame that comes with the territory of being childless in our culture right now and it's important that you question it. It's a place where your Inner Bitch can take up residence, pushing you forward into projects and places that *look* meaningful but which are actually just more ways for you to prove to yourself and to others that you matter, *even though you're not a mother.*

This is subtle bullshit and you'll need a subtle bullshit detector to find it. Here are a few questions to ask yourself:

- If the results from doing this were invisible, could I be bothered to do it?
- Would I do it even if I didn't get paid for it?
- Would I do it even if no one ever knew about it?
- Who am I doing it for?

Whilst meaning is the lifebuoy in the stormy seas of childlessness, you don't need to make a grab for each flotation device that comes into view – you just need the one with *your* name on it. And finding that 'one' may require some experimentation. It may be that you need to do a few 'big' things before you work out that you don't have the energy for them and that they're just not for you. That's not a failure – that's feedback.

> You don't need a big life on the outside to be a happily childless woman; but you *do* need a big life on the *inside*.

Being a childless woman in our motherhood-crazy world can feel like as much of a 'full time job' as being a mother. It's just that the work is internal, invisible and involves a constant pushing-back against the deluge of messages that there's something wrong with us, that we're not welcome, that we've failed. Not being crushed and deformed by those messages – that is our life's work. And we'll get no credit from others for it, unlike the endless public plaudits of motherhood. As a result, we often don't even give ourselves credit for it.

Whether your Plan B ends up looking ordinary, extraordinary or maybe a bit of both is up to you. It's about whatever kind of love affair with life works for you.

We are reluctant pioneers – we didn't choose to be so different, but now that we are, we have the chance to shape and create a life that feels meaningful to us. And to us alone.

EXERCISE 16: YOUR FIRST PLAN B

Turn off the phone, lock the door, turn off the radio, feed the cat – do whatever you need to get total peace and privacy for about an hour.

Get yourself some paper and pens, or a special notebook. Create a template of the 6 Human Needs using the instructions from earlier in the chapter. If you like to draw things – take a lovely drawing pad and colours. Hell, get the glitter pens, Post-It notes, scissors, fluffy pompoms and gold stars out! When I do a similar exercise in workshops, everyone looks very nervous when I get all these fun things out, yet by the end everything gets used and a lot of fun is had. You'll also need a timer. Maybe get a glass of wine, or light a candle. This is meant to be enjoyable.

Sit down in a chair, or on the floor, in the garden – wherever you are most comfortable, and spend a couple of minutes breathing gently and relaxing.

When you are peaceful and comfortable, set the timer for ten minutes. You're going to do a visualisation exercise.

Close your eyes and imagine a day in your life about five years hence, when your Plan B is rocking along and you're living a life of meaning, purpose and connection. You're happy and fulfilled and no longer crushed by your childlessness. Life has worked out amazingly well, all things considered, and you can't quite believe your luck.

Let yourself daydream about this day, as if it were happening today. Be playful – this is a daydream after all. Imagine how you'd feel, look, be, behave...

- What clothes are you wearing?
- What's happening in your life that day?
- What will already have taken place and be in your life on that day?
- What kind of people are around you?
- What is your environment like?
- What does it look like, smell like, feel like, sound like?
- Look off into the distance - what can you see?

Let yourself daydream like you did when you were a child and allow yourself to drift away into this new place...

And then, when the timer goes off... capture it, in whatever way feels most like you:

- Quickly write it all down. Write it in the present tense, as if it were happening today, right now. And whatever you do, don't edit anything out as being stupid or impossible. Not yet: this is play.

- If it's easier for you, or as an experiment, you might want to talk it all into the 'speech recorder' function on your phone if you have one.

- Have a go at drawing what you've seen – that's where the glitter pens come in! Remember this is play and no one needs to see this but you.

Once you feel you've captured it, see if you can map your vision onto the 6 Human Needs template and see how different parts of it satisfy different Human Needs. This is still fantasy, try not to let your sensible head start editing yet…

Starting really, really, small, for now, choose one element of your vision to put into action. Baby steps, that's the idea.

> Your first Plan B is *not* about committing yourself to a course of action that's going to last the rest of your life.

It needs to be an element that has a positive charge for you, something that gives you a sweet flutter inside that's somewhere between fear and excitement. Nothing worthy or sensible – for example if losing weight or getting a new job have been on your 'to do' list for ages this isn't what you're looking for. However, if in your visualisation you were accepting an award for garden design and you love gardening but have never thought you could make a living from it, that's something with a 'positive charge'.

Now, before you start yelling at me that it's not realistic, not possible, can't afford it, what kind of crazy-arsed book is this… STOP!! *I'm not saying, 'go and do it.' I'm asking you to let yourself have a daydream!*

It's not about selling your house, buying a VW camper van and moving to Nova Scotia to study rare birds. In fact, I strongly recommend that you *avoid* doing anything you can't change your mind about. Baby steps, remember – not *huge* decisions.

What did you want to be when you grew up? A ballerina, a spy, a vet, a nurse, a pop star, a doctor, an explorer? Do you still want to? Probably not. You had other dreams that came later.

And so it'll be with your first Plan B. The fact is you're probably out of practice with imagining new possibilities, so I recommend that you keep your training-wheels on for a while. Try out a few low-risk ideas and as your identity as someone who's washed-up and can't change evolves into something new, your Plan B will evolve along with it.

So what's the lowest risk, most fun (it has to be fun!) thing you can do in the next week to try out an element of your daydream Plan B? *Go do it.* It can be whatever tickles your fancy:

- Walking through the doors of the art college you've been going past on your way to work and wishing you'd gone there 20 years earlier – just to smell the air and pick up a prospectus.
- Writing a poem about looking for your Plan B.
- Finding your sewing machine under the pile of 'must do mending' and making something just for fun.
- Going beach-combing as part of a garden project, or maybe because you have a hankering to become a geologist…
- Signing up for the open evening at your local choir because you used to love singing.
- Heading to the zoo with your sketchbook.

- Cooking a new recipe for that cake shop you fantasise about.
- Doing some hula-hooping, roller-skating, ice-skating – anything that feels like fun and that you don't do because you don't have kids.
- Getting creative with your wardrobe again.
- And there's nothing wrong with researching whether there *are* any campervans for sale and what qualifications you *might* need to work as a rare breed conservationist specialising in eagles. As long as you also *do* something, like go birdwatching.

You just have to take that first baby step. It all starts with that first step. Self-esteem is built by keeping our promises to ourselves – so it's really important that you start following through. Which is why it's really important to make it genuinely something you really want to do, not too difficult or expensive and *definitely* not too sensible.

Your Plan B starts when you do, and where it might end up – who knows? It's an adventure, your adventure. Which is good, because on their deathbed nobody wishes they'd spent more time at the office…

REFLECTIONS ON THIS CHAPTER

In this chapter, we've been looking at creating some of the elements that might become part of your first Plan B – your first baby steps towards creating a meaningful and fulfilling life without children. Ultimately, it doesn't matter what your Plan B is – it's whatever works for you. One woman's life of meaning is another woman's 'Meh'.

*Although you may have initially been a bit disappointed that I didn't solve your Plan B dilemma, I also hope that you understand that **no answer I could give you** would ever really wash. That only **you** know what makes your wings itch to fly again, only **you** have the skills to make it happen.*

*Did you find time to follow through on your baby step or did you find reasons not to do so? Sometimes, taking that first step can be surprisingly hard, so if you found it difficult, it might be that it just wasn't fun enough. You may have given yourself something else to add to your 'to do list'… and that won't do at all! This first step needs to be something you're absolutely **busting** to do, if only you'd let yourself do it. To get your Plan B going, you're going to need to learn to start experimenting with your life again – so don't see this as a failure, but as feedback to help guide you as you learn what lights your fire. This is not a one-shot deal.*

And if you did take that baby step, how was it? Was it as hard as you thought it was going to be or was it actually a bit too easy? Perhaps now you've taken that step, you're ready to take a slightly bigger one. This is the beginning of a journey back to ourselves and sometimes it's easier than we think – we just need to give ourselves permission and to seek out and allow some encouragement. We need our tribe.

Although we are now coming towards the end of this book, you stand at the threshold of a whole new beginning. Take a moment to acknowledge how far you've come and make some plans to celebrate when you get to the end of Chapter 12. We have so few rituals as childless women, separated as we are from those of family life – so get together with other NoMos and have a ball!

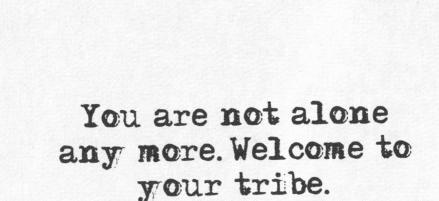

You are **not** alone
any more. Welcome to
your tribe.

CHAPTER 12

TAKING OFF THE INVISIBILITY CLOAK

WELCOME TO YOUR TRIBE

My first thought when I found out that 1:5 women were turning 45 without having had children was this: *Well where the hell are they all then?!*

Before I started Gateway Women I was, amongst all my friends and colleagues over the years, as far as I know, the only woman who wanted a child and didn't get to have one. I knew a couple of women who chose not have children, but none who longed for motherhood and had had to come to terms with it never happening. I felt so isolated in my situation, like I was the only one.

I've spoken to enough childless women now to know that my isolation is quite a common experience. After all, if four out of five women are mothers, the chances of being the 'only one' who's childless in your family and social group must be quite high.

Amongst those women several years younger than me and born in the 1970s however, there seem to be many more who increasingly worry that motherhood isn't going to happen for them. All of them for reasons of 'social infertility' – in that they have been unable so far to find a suitable partner to settle down and raise a family with and time is running out. Very few of them either want or can afford to become 'solo mothers' by choice.

However, if you turn on the TV, watch movies, follow celebrity gossip, read women's magazines or pay attention to how products aimed at women are marketed, you wouldn't think there was any woman alive who wasn't dating, engaged, trying to conceive, pregnant, married, a mother or a grandmother. And as for women without children over the age of 40, we're almost completely absent from any kind of cultural representation.

> Now, I don't know about you, but I haven't been through what I've been through to become invisible!

We looked at some of the cultural and historical reasons as to why this might be in Chapter 5, but what I'm interested in here is thinking about what we can do to *change* the record. We have a great deal to offer to our communities, our culture and the wider world. However, before we can get others to realise this we first need to realise it *ourselves*. Each one of us that reclaims our self-esteem and lives a life of meaning makes a difference. We don't have to woman the barricades, just living our lives unapologetically and publicly is all that's needed – just as gay men and women have learned to do. Because:

- We can be a huge force for good in this world at a time when the world has probably never been more in need of it.

- We are women whose hearts have been broken by life but who have had the courage to heal ourselves and move forward. That makes us fabulous role models.

- We are brave, wise, independent, educated, aware, soulful, compassionate women who just happen not to have children.

- We are the NoMos (the not-mothers). Individually we're impressive. Collectively, we're awesome.

It's time we removed the invisibility cloak and showed the world what we're made of. Stereotypes can be changed, one woman at a time.

Imagine how different it would have been for you if you had known of *other* women who'd come to terms with their childlessness and had gone on to create a life of meaning? Imagine if such women were a part of the culture – seen on TV and in magazines as normal people, not 'cautionary tales' or 'freaks', but just as another way to be an adult woman?

Just imagine that for a moment. Let it sink in. Think how much easier it would have been.

Each one of us who has the courage to feel OK about ourselves, despite the messages we're getting from the culture, is a heroine. We don't need to be Mother Teresa or Oprah to do this. Just being ourselves and refusing to feel ashamed is all that we need to do to start changing things.

However, it may be simple, but it won't be easy. As Gloria Steinem wrote in 1971:

> *Any woman who chooses to behave like a full human being should be warned that the armies of the status quo will treat her as something of a dirty joke. That's their natural and first weapon. She will need her sisterhood.*[71]

NoMos: your world needs you, as do all the young women coming of age in a world without role models of what happy, fulfilled lives as childless-by-circumstance women might look like.

Building Your Tribe

Finding a way to be with other childless women who are exploring, embracing or rocking their Plan B is just about the best thing you can do to make yourself feel visible again. It's transformed my life and I love watching the process of transformation happen for other women too.

In the Gateway Women groups and workshops I see women arrive tightly buttoned up, nervous and shaky, ready to bolt for the door at any minute. Gradually I see them soften and open as the session unfolds. I see a look somewhere between disbelief and relief on their faces as they hear parts of their *own* story coming out of *another* woman's mouth. I watch them let go of their fear of being open about their situation as they realise that, perhaps, for the first time, no one's going to say: 'It's OK, you've still loads of time' or, 'You could still adopt' or, 'Women of 50 are having babies now' or any of the other hundred well-meaning sentences that we dread after hearing them so many times.

I watch the women in the room look around and come to admire and identify with other women as they realise that they are not alone in having been brought to their knees by their childlessness. I notice their thinking begin to shift as they begin to realise that maybe, after all, it's not *all their own fault.*

Then come the tears and the laughter as they work together to tease out hidden prejudices, to share their shame and watch it evaporate, to tentatively start forgiving themselves, their bodies, their choices, their fortunes and watch as new friendships form based on trust, respect and shared experience.

Women start arriving early and leaving late. They start meeting up outside the groups and workshops. They do their homework eagerly, they report breakthroughs, they start looking different, wearing different clothes and brighter colours. They report new and startling insights and conversations.

And then, solidarity, sisterhood, a tribal bond. They come to understand that they're not alone, not freaks. Careers are reassessed, creative projects are taken up again, nieces and nephews are embraced with affection not desperation, partners and parents are let off the hook. They start taking responsibility for their own happiness again.

> They say it takes a whole village to raise a child. Well, I think it takes a whole tribe to heal a childless woman. Gateway Women is that tribe.

If you're feeling isolated in your childlessness I can guarantee that there are other women in your town also sitting at home feeling marooned in a sea of mothers. You are not weird and you are not alone. You're 1:5 women turning 45. Find a way to connect with your tribe and it all starts to get a lot easier. Maybe even, dare I say it, *fun* again…

STOP TRYING TO STAY YOUNG

Whatever age you are today, all of us are going to be childless older women in the future. And, as none of the current stereotypes for childless older women is designed to make us feel good, this can make the idea of being comfortable in our skins as we age quite problematic! (See more on this in Chapter 5).

In some ways, the current cultural cult of unending youth and the fetishisation of motherhood are both ways of denying what comes after: the elder woman – what used to be called the 'crone'. The crone was as feared as she was revered – and yes, she could be a grumpy old woman as well as a wise and kindly old soul. Crones are human too – not fairy godmothers.

After all we've lived through and all we've endured and with maternal hearts that long to give to others, why *should* we damn well go quietly into the night?

> We have scars on our hearts but fire in our souls so who gives a damn if we don't look young anymore?

Hello – we're *not* young anymore and as soon as *we* stop having a problem with that or giving any headspace to the fact that *others* might have a problem with us still being here, things will get better for all women.

I go along with a quotation widely attributed to from Hunter S. Thompson on this one:

> *Life should not be a journey to the grave with the intention of arriving in a pretty and well preserved body, but rather to skid in broadside, thoroughly used up, totally worn out, and loudly proclaiming, 'Wow, what a ride!'*

If as intelligent, powerful older women we spend our time worrying about our looks, chasing after a vanished youth or lying about our age we are, in effect, participating in our own shaming, our own invisibility.

It is precisely *because* we don't have children, just as it was for many of the old healers and midwives, that we have the time to pursue knowledge for its own sake and to make shifts happen in our own lives and in the culture. How many of us have advanced degrees in more than one area, and are pursuing the love of learning for just that – love? How many of us train for second careers that we are passionate about when we finally accept that we are never going to be mothers? How many of us have an enviable sparkle in our eyes that no cosmetic 'work' can match because we've done the *internal* work to get our mojo working again?

What an asset we can be to the next generation if only we realise it and claim it. Hey, most people think we're invisible, so we can make all kinds of stuff happen before anyone's going to realise what we're up to!

The time has come to take our place in society as powerful older women with opinions that matter. Young women are too inexperienced and preoccupied with dating and mating, mothers with young children are too busy and our wonderful men are exhausted and running out of ideas. It's time to rebalance the culture before it's too late and integrate the wisdom of the older women (both mothers *and* NoMos) back into our world.

Only when masculine and feminine work hand in hand will we be able to create a fairer world for all. That's what feminism ultimately is about – equal rights, equal responsibility. It's not, as many fear, about a new matriarchy. We owe it to the generations that follow us, even if they're not our children, to leave things better than we found them.

> We are the grown-ups – it's time we started acting like it and not running around worrying about our age, the sizes of our arses or what other people think of us.

Never before in recorded history have so many women like us been alive at the same time: intelligent, liberated, educated, financially-independent women not involved in bringing up children. And never has the western world seemed so in need of an injection of wise, compassionate, heart-felt thinking. If we NoMos collectively realised our power, imagine how different things could be?

If we NoMos collectively realised our power, imagine how different things could be?

However, perhaps one of the single biggest fears that's holding us back from claiming that power is our fear of old age and what that might hold for us.

Old Lady Blues

Perhaps one of the most pernicious fears of childless women, particularly single childless women, is who's going to take care of us when we're old. Even in our modern world, children are still seen as the answer to old age.

> I've come to realise that it's not that children *are* the answer to an adult's care needs when they're elderly, but that having children gives parents the luxury of not thinking through these difficult issues. As childless women, we don't have that fantasy – we have to face the music.

Being old is a taboo in our society, obsessed as it is with youth, with control, with personal power and agency. The lack of obvious carers for elderly childless women brings every adult's unspoken fear out in the open. But rather than accept that this is an issue that everyone will face, a lot of the fear is projected back onto childless women. Some research into 'Ageing Without Children' that I participated in conducted by Dr Mary Pat Sullivan from Brunel University and Dr Mo Ray of Keele University in 2013 found that in fact the outcomes for single, childless elderly men are far more troubling.[72]

It's time to explore and explode a few of these fears and myths that surround growing old without children:

Myth 1: Having children guarantees that you will be taken care of when you're old

- Now, many children (including ourselves) do indeed take care of their parent's needs when old, but it's not a guarantee…

- OK. First and most brutal question – how are you and your siblings (if you have any) getting on with your parents?

- Do you have plans to have your elderly parent(s) come and

live with you when they need to? Do you have room for them physically and emotionally?

- Even if your relationship with your parents is very good, the reality is that it may be logistically impossible for you to give them a home in their old age. You may live on the other side of the country or world, or in a one-room flat that you're already stretched financially to afford. Our generation does not have the cushion of rising property values and great pensions that the Boomers had.

- Also, who knows, you may die before your parents...

- So, if you had had children, why would they too not have been subject to the same issues?

Myth 2: Having children guarantees grandchildren to keep you company in your old age and bring some joy into your life

Many grandparents do enjoy the company of their grandchildren and find that they bring them joy, but it's not a guarantee ...

- What if you'd had children and they didn't have children – we of all people should know it's not a given!

- Your grandchildren might have ended up living on the other side of the world.

- You might not have liked your grandchildren very much or might have fallen out with their parents over the values they were bringing them up with.

- You might have found yourself having to be your grandchildren's primary carer whilst their parents worked full time and so what you had hoped was going to be a bit of joy once a week turned into an exhausting 8am-8pm job.

- You might have enough joy in your own life by then anyway! Who says only grandchildren can bring a sparkle to your eyes?

There's every chance that, with your Plan B (or Plan X, Y or Z) rocking along, *you'll* be the one bringing joy into your own life and possibly into many others too!

- If you have children and young people in your life now who care about you (nephews, nieces, godchildren, young colleagues, mentees, friends' children) there's no reason to suppose that one or more of them might not be your ally in old age. They might even want to do it, rather than feel that they have to, because you're someone they love, cherish and admire and you've been a great mentor and role model to them of a life well lived.

Myth 3: *You will be a helpless, senile old woman*

- Whilst old age does mean a decline in vitality, an unhealthy old age is not a given. A healthy lifestyle and an active mind *now* could make all the difference *then*. And a positive attitude and joyful heart can make it possible to have a happy old age even with unavoidable infirmities. We know, from our experience of childlessness, that the way we *think* about our situation is as important as the situation itself in how we cope with it. In fact, we're probably *better* equipped than many of our childed peers to deal with the changes and challenges of old age.

- The Boomer generation, now just entering into old age, has changed everything it's passed through – relationships, education, work, love, parenting and spirituality. They're going to change 'old age' too. We're frightening ourselves with an old-fashioned idea of being elderly.

- Retirement is a phrase that will sound very quaint in generations to come – it's an unaffordable luxury for many and the changing demographics and life-expectancy of our generation mean that quite a few of us will be on our third

Plan B by the time we're of 'pensionable age'. Get your Plan B going now and you stand every chance of being a busy, connected and involved elder woman. I think perhaps the women who may have a tougher time than us are those mothers who get divorced in their 50s once their children have left home and have little idea how to navigate the new working landscape. Our resourcefulness and knowledge learned from navigating a life without the identity of motherhood may become priceless as we move into old age.

- Care for the elderly is an issue that our generation needs to address before it's too late (well, it's already too late, but that's usually when things get done!) It needs to be sorted out for everyone – because, even for those who *do* have children, those children cannot be relied upon to have the time, inclination or resources to take care of their elderly parents for 20 years. How a culture treats its most vulnerable members is a telling mark of how 'civilised' it really is. Elderly care is an issue that our culture needs to face, and face without flinching. Our elders are precious, not rubbish to be put out.

Myth 4: *You will be a lonely old woman*

- Some old women are great fun, appear to have a wide circle of friends, enjoy going to funerals to see their friends and are great at making new friends in new situations. If that's what you're like as a person now (minus the funeral hopping, I hope) you'll hopefully still be like that as an old woman. I'm definitely less gregarious than I was in my 20s and 30s, yet I'm much more confident and the warmth that used to be hidden under a brittle surface of bravado is now much more visible, which makes it easier for people to get to know me. I'm good at connecting with new people, good at keeping up with technology and I'm getting used to the fact that as a childless woman it's usually up to me to reach out and make new connections. Sometimes it gets a bit wearing, doing it all without the 'school gate' club, but that's what organisations like Gateway Women are for – a new tribe, a different set of 'gates'.

- Loneliness is a part of life and it isn't to be feared if we have developed a good relationship with ourselves and with our spirit, our source. If we outlive our partner or don't have one and maybe outlive or are geographically distanced from our friends, there will probably be times of loneliness in later life. However, if we reorient 'loneliness' as 'solitude' and welcome it as a time to go deeper within, we don't need to fear it. A fear of loneliness is, ultimately, a fear of ourselves. Boredom is different – and hopefully we will have created such a rich life by then, full of meaning, that we won't have the time to be bored. I don't mean to downplay how crushing isolation feels – I've experienced it and would never belittle it. But it taught me a lot about myself and I faced and survived a really primal human fear.

- One of the best antidotes to loneliness I know is *giving*. It makes a connection that I think gives more to the giver than the receiver, although the receiver hopefully gets a lot out of it too! As big-hearted women who longed to be mothers we have a lot to give and it's vital that we find a way to keep doing so as we grow old. Whether it's by being involved in our local community or the wider world, we can *always* find a way to contribute and we *must* do so in order to feel connected. There are always ways to give of ourselves; we *always* have something to offer.

- As childless women we know what it is to live on the margins of society, and many of us have already suffered from ostracism, isolation and loneliness. We know what it is to feel that we are 'wrong', and 'defective' and not to be able to avoid our sense of being alone in a vast universe by throwing ourselves into family life and the identity of motherhood. As a result we're possibly *better* prepared for the falling away of familiar support, social structures, friends and family that so often accompanies advanced old age than some other people. We *know* that we need a strong network of like-minded, psychologically mature, emotionally generous and spiritually competent people to keep us sane and safe – and so we put time into building and sustaining those relationships. There is no reason to suppose that the skills it takes to make, honour and sustain networks will be any different in our old age. And, unlike our own grandparents, we will also be able to reach out and keep in touch via the Internet and video-conferencing services. If you're someone who is resistant to computers, this might be the time to change your mind whilst you're still young enough to become competent. You cannot afford your technophobia anymore – the price it may cost you later may be shockingly high.

Myth 5: *You will die alone*

- Anyone can die alone. It's a very human fear and to a great extent it's out of our control. I hope that my friends who have children do indeed get to spend their last days and moments with their children beside them, but it can't be guaranteed.

- Think about this: if you were to die in a month's time, would you die alone or would you die surrounded by friends and family wishing you well on your journey? In that case, why do you think that the person you're going to be in 20 or 30 years is going to have such a different experience? When you think of yourself as an old woman, don't you realise that the person you're imagining isn't someone else – she's you! If you have friends and family who love you now, are you planning to fall out and lose touch with every single one of them by then and not make any new close connections between now and the time you die? Don't you think that at least one of your nephews, nieces, godchildren, students, young colleagues or young friends might be around to sit with you, even if everyone else your own age has died? When you actually think about it, the fear of dying alone because you don't have children is a very human fear, and no more likely for us than for most people. We live in an atomised, global world: it could happen to anyone, not just us. And perhaps, because we're a little less smug about our children being there for us, we might actually make a bit more preparation, and take better care of our friendships, just in case… Which can't be a bad thing, can it?

- This is a slightly utopian vision, but I'm wondering if one of the things we could do as NoMos is to start planning a way of living in a community as we get older – the Gateway Village. In my mind's eye it's a cross between a yoga retreat, a university of the third age and a retirement community. It would be our own gathering of elders where we could continue to support and amuse each other, whilst carrying on cooking up trouble till the day we kick the bucket. Because we don't fit in we don't *have* to. We can do what we want. We can make the rules and break the rules. We can have old age on our own terms, and create somewhere and something compassionate, adventurous and caring.

THINKING ABOUT YOUR LEGACY

For some of us, thinking about a legacy means thinking about to whom we are going to leave our money and possessions when we die. However, there's another form of legacy that's particularly important for childless women and that's thinking about what we leave behind. What footprint our life leaves on this earth.

A life well lived is a precious thing, and the lessons learned in that life deserve to be passed on in some way. I often feel that having been denied the opportunity to pass our values, stories and wisdom on to our children or grandchildren is another invisible loss that we have to grieve. However, there are other ways that we can celebrate and pass on our wisdom.

It might be that some of us, as we get older, find ways to contribute to our community and to the following generations, although, as with everything we do, we'll have to make it happen. There are no 'traditions' for us to step into.

Some examples of a legacy might be:

- A special relationship with a young person to whom you act as a mentor.

- A skill that you pass on.

- Your example as someone who has transformed pain into growth and came out of it with wisdom rather than bitterness.

- Your creative outputs: a book, a play, a painting, a garden, a business, an idea.

- A change in the way the younger generation in your extended family and community think about childlessness and their options.

- Your part in the NoMo movement.

- Etc.

In the past, elders in the culture were valued as a source of wisdom. Indeed, in some Native American cultures it is believed that when a woman stops menstruating, her blood is retained inside her as wisdom instead. They also have a tradition that *all* elder women are known as 'grandmothers', whether mothers or not and all are treated with respect and revered for their knowledge and wisdom. This tradition continues in more traditional societies such as some parts of the southern Mediterranean.

> Can you imagine how much wisdom we'll have about how to create a life of meaning by the time we are old women? Does it seem sensible or acceptable that this knowledge is not passed on?

However, before we get too carried away we need to remember that, in Western culture, ancestors are not revered down the generations. Indeed, how well do you know your own family history beyond that of your own grandparent's generation? It is the fate of most of us to be forgotten by history, whether we have children or not. Yes, some exceptional individuals do leave their mark on history, but just because we're childless, we don't have to force ourselves to be one of them. That'll be the Inner Bitch again!

We Are the Role Models

If I had known that a happy and fulfilling life without children was possible, I might have begun the process of accepting my situation much earlier than I did. But when the alternative to motherhood looked so bleak that I couldn't even contemplate it, what choice did I have but to just keep on hoping, keep on planning, keep on dreaming and keep putting my life on hold in my quest to become a mother? Even just one role model of a woman I admired who was childless-by-circumstance and had found a way forward would have made a massive difference to me.

There are very few positive role models of childless women who spring to mind and, of those that do, many of them will be childfree-by-choice rather than childless-by-circumstance.

You may have noticed that when a woman in the public eye has children, she talks about them, even if it's to say that she *doesn't* talk about them. Yet, if she's a childless woman and past childbearing age, the topic is considered unmentionable. It's off limits, taboo. Unless that individual woman chooses to talk about it, we are completely in the dark about her story – whether she's childfree or if she's ended up without children for one of the many complicated reasons that *we* all know so well. She's usually labelled with a stereotype (career woman, lesbian, unfeminine, etc.) and *her* side of the story is rarely heard or sought. The invisibility cloak goes on and that's that, case closed.

If childless-by-circumstance women *do* get media attention, it's often to be pitied or to be sold yet another 'miracle baby story' about a woman in her 50s who's given birth, reinforcing the notion that we should 'never give up'. But what does that say about its alternative – coming to terms with childlessness? It says it's either not possible or that it has no value.

> Just as we as individuals find change hard, so does society. The change is happening, and the media and culture will reflect that, in time.

It seems that our current place is to be either a sob story or a miracle baby story with not much in-between. This isn't helped by the fact that it's often a real challenge to get women other than me to contribute publicly to stories in the media because they feel too ashamed to be named. That's where we are today, but it will change – it's already changing and I curate a 'board' on Pinterest of more than 250 childless and childfree women role models.[73] As more and more of us get the support to do our grief work and start working on our Plan Bs, the invisibility cloaks will be dropped. As more and more of us put down the burden of shame society says is our lot, things will change.

Coming to terms with childlessness is hard, but it's worth it. After all, we've tried the alternative... It's vital, if future generations of women are not to suffer in silence as we have done, that we live our Plan Bs as unapologetically and frankly as possible.

It is only by refusing to be ashamed that the taboo of shame will be broken.

Some of the things that need to come out in the open are:

- Talking about our childlessness and the impact it's had on our lives without shame, or apologising for ourselves. We have a right to be sad. We have a right to our stories – including positive ones about creating a meaningful and fulfilling life without children.

- Getting the message out there that IVF is not a magic bullet and that more women and couples come out of fertility treatments *without* a family than the media coverage of miracle babies would suggest. The starker reality is that IVF is frontier science and in 2012 had a global failure rate of 77%.[74]

- Teenagers need to be taught about fertility as well as contraception to avoid the notion that getting pregnant later in life is 'easy'.

- To challenge the current thinking that makes the idea of having a family in your 20s and pursuing further education and a career later so unacceptable. If we're all going to live till we're almost 100 years old and work till the day we die, what's the rush?

- To challenge the social and political structures that make it so hard for professional women and couples to be able to combine careers and childrearing.

- To bridge the gap between mothers and NoMos by showing that although our life experience is different, in a long life, our solidarity as women is more important.

- We need to finish the work that the sexual revolution began and make both men *and* women, both parents *and* non-parents, equally of value in our culture.

- There are many other things we need to speak out about – how we are treated by our families, friends, employers, communities and our governments being just a short list of a big task!

> It is not necessary to be an activist in a stereotypical way: simply by living our lives openly and refusing to be shamed by our circumstance we are role models.

Childlessness is not the end of our story. It's the start of a new way of life, the life unexpected. And there's no reason why our new lives can't rock, in our own way, to our own tune.

Go sister, go!

APPENDIX

Contents:

- **Plan B Healing Inventory** – complete this before and after working through this book, or whenever you wish. You will also find a downloadable copy of this on the Gateway Women website at www.gateway-women.com

- **Online Resources** – blogs, websites, forums and other resources from around the world for childless-by-circumstance women. Included in the online resource list at bit.ly/1ca5jEN

- **Recommended Reading** – books that I've read and which have supported me, and others, as we heal from our childlessness and move towards our Plan B. Included in the online resource list at bit.ly/1ca5jEN

- **Acknowledgements** – a thank you to all of you who have helped make this book possible.

PLAN B HEALING INVENTORY

Your Name:

Today's Date:

Your Age:

Please score the following questions on a scale of 0 to 10 (where 0 is 'not much' and 10 is 'a lot')

1. How easy do you find it being around your friends and family's children?

2. How easy do you find it to talk to people about your situation and history?

3. How bothered are you by people asking you if you have kids?

4. How comfortable are you holding a baby in your arms?

5. How much do you believe that there are other ways to experience the joy, connection and meaning in life that mothers seem to have?

6. How angry are you about how things have turned out?

7. How much shame or embarrassment do you feel about your situation or history?

8. How much do you blame other people for how things have turned out?

9. How sad are you about how things have turned out?

10. How much do you enjoy the benefits that come with not having children?

11. How bothered are you with how people may perceive you as a childless woman?

12. How aware are you of inspiring childless-by-circumstance women role models?

13. How strong is your mojo these days?

14. How full of clutter is your home?

15. How comfortable are you with the idea of taking risks and doing things differently?

16. How often do you really laugh your head off these days?

17. How willing are you to let go of the dream of motherhood?

18. How often do you pleasantly daydream about your childless future?

19. How often do you worry about your childless future?

20. How well do you take care of your body?

21. How happy are you with the way you look?

22. How connected to your inner world do you feel?

23. How kind are you to yourself?

24. How much of a bitch are you to yourself?

25. How nurturing and 'mothering' is your inner dialogue?

26. How much do you enjoy your work?

27. How much do you feel like an 'outsider' in your workplace or with colleagues?

28. How creative do you think you are?

29. How much play is there in your daily life?

30. How strong is your physical health for your age?

31. How many minor illnesses do you get?

32. How much do you believe that you're capable of finding a Plan B?

33. How much of you is scared that you're uniquely equipped to fail at life?

34. How important is meaning to you?

35. How much do you worry about growing old without children?

36. How much importance do you give to leaving a legacy?

37. How much do you believe that you personally are capable of making a contribution to this world other than by being a mother?

38. How connected, stimulated and supported do you feel by your current social circle?

39. How happy are you to be alive?

40. How ready are you to rock the life unexpected?

Online Resources

- **Gateway Women website (Global)**

  www.gateway-women.com

  Jody Day's Gateway Women website full of articles and resources for childless-by-circumstance women. UK based, global audience.

- **Gateway Women Private Online Community on G+ (Global)**

  To apply for membership of the 'best online community for childless-by-circumstance women' (that's a review, not me!) go to www.gateway-women.com and click on 'Online Community'. All applications are vetted for member security and privacy.

- **Gateway Women Meetup Group (UK / Global)**

  www.meetup.com/gateway-women

  Private Meetup group for childless-by-circumstance women who wish to meet up in person. UK based, with members from UK, USA, Canada and Australia.

- **Gateway Women Resource Centre on Listly (Global)**

  http://list.ly/l/13P

  An online library of articles and resources of relevance to childless-by-circumstance women from online resources globally. At the last count over 300 articles and resources. Browse and feel free to add your own too as you come across them and let's curate the web collaboratively.

- **Gateway Women Gallery of Childless & Childfree Role Models on Pinterest (Global)**

  http://pinterest.com/gatewaywomen/gateway-women-childless-childfree-women-role-model/

  Or bit.ly/13fQUBw if you need to type it in!

  Portraits and mini-biographies of childless and childfree women role models. 250+ women from different cultures and times, with more being added as I hear about them. Take a look and suggest your own too by becoming a Pinner to this board.

- **Childless Stepmothers (UK)**

  www.childlessstepmums.co.uk

  Being a stepmother can be very challenging, being a childless stepmother uniquely so. This UK-based internet forum describes itself as 'a sanctuary for women thrown into an instant family of often angry ex-wives, resentful stepchildren and guilty or mourning fathers'.

- **The Daisy Network (UK)**

  www.daisynetwork.org.uk

  A UK charity that supports women who have experienced premature menopause or premature ovarian failure as it's often referred to.

- **From Forty With Love (UK)**

  www.fromfortywithlove.com

  A blog by British journalist Katherine Baldwin about being 40+, single & still hopeful of having a family and how this came about. Although Katherine is not in the 'Plan B' camp, her writing and thinking around ambivalence is something that many of us can relate to.

- **More to Life (UK)**

  www.infertilitynetworkuk.com/more_to_life

  A UK charity that provides online and face-to-face groups for women and couples moving on after infertility treatment.

- **Childless by Marriage (US)**

  www.childlessbymarriage.blogspot.com.au

  Writer and musician Sue Fagalde Lick's book and blog about life as a childless stepmother and now as a childless widow living on her own.

- **Childless Mothers Connect (CMC) and Childless Mothers Adopt (CMomA) (US)**

  www.cmoma.org/cmc

  Psychotherapist Dr Marcy Cole's website, organisation and community for 'Childless Mothers' (by both choice and circumstance) and her project (CMomA) to connect children-in-need with adoptive or foster mothers. Marcy is a childless-by-circumstance woman herself.

- **Chopra Center (US)**

  bit.ly/16lLMOV

  Free downloads of guided meditations by Davidji.

  If you're new to meditation, these short guided meditations by Davidji are a great place to start. Davidji is a warm, real and very experienced Californian meditation teacher with a lovely voice. I'm very fussy so I think you'll like these!

  www.chopra.com
  www.davidji.com

- **Life Without Baby (US)**

  www.lifewithoutbaby.com

  Lisa Manterfield's blog, online community, online courses & resources for women coming to terms with life as a childless woman. Lisa is the author of 'I'm Taking my Eggs and Going Home'.

- **Savvy Auntie (US)**

  www.savvyauntie.com

  www.huffingtonpost.com/melanie-notkin

  Melanie Notkin's US site for women without children who are aunts, godmothers or in some way 'childful'. Also has a busy online community. Melanie Notkin also writes movingly for Huffington Post on being a single, childless woman in her mid-40s.

- **The Bitter Babe (US)**

  www.thebitterbabe.wordpress.com

  An anonymous blog charting the outer and inner life of a forty-something single childless woman. Frank, insightful and culturally astute, this is the very best writing I've seen on the issue from a personal, sociological and cultural viewpoint. I hope she writes a book soon!

- **Listening Earth (AUS)**

  www.listeningearth.com

  A library of high-quality nature recordings from around the world made by a couple without children for whom this is their life's passion. Read the blog – they have an amazing life doing what they love. You can sample the tracks before you download or purchase the CDs. I recommend you have a listen to the recordings closest in sound to the environment where you spent your earliest years – for example, rainforest sounds make me jumpy, but British birdsong calms me!

RECOMMENDED READING

Some of these books are out of print, but if so, you can often get a second-hand copy from www.abebooks.co.uk or www.amazon.co.uk or read them in e-book form. All the 'bitly' links will take you to the Google Book entry rather than a bookstore where you can often read a free extract to see if you'd like to purchase the book.

For those books with the word 'God' in the title or with content in them that refers to God or other faiths – in my opinion, these books are suitable for readers of all faiths or none.

All these books are also listed online as part of the Listly List for this book bit.ly/1aeMuMp

Links which start with 'bit.ly' are shortened versions of much longer links in case you have to type them in rather than click them.

On social & cultural aspects of childlessness-by-circumstance

- Cain, M. (2001) *The Childless Revolution: What It Means to be a Childless Woman Today.* New York: Persus Books

  A good general reader's overview of the factors and stories behind the increase in women without children – by choice, chance and 'happenstance'.

  bit.ly/179MYCs

  www.madelyncain.com

- Cannold, L. (2005) *What, No Baby? Why women are losing the freedom to mother and how they can get it back.* Freemantle, Australia: Curtin University Books.

  The best-written and most thoroughly researched book on the subject I've read. Suitable for both the academic and general reader.

  bit.ly/12vUa7t

  www.cannold.com

- Carroll, L. (2012) *The Baby Matrix: Why Freeing Our Minds from Outmoded Thinking About Parenting and Reproduction Will Create a Better World.* USA: LiveTrue Books

  An excellent and very provocative book that blows the lid off pronatalism and suggests really interesting alternative ways of thinking and behaving around having/not having children.

  bit.ly/1budgmc
  www.lauracarroll.com

On midlife and growing older without children

- Athill, D. (2009) *Somewhere Towards The End.* UK: Granta Books.

  Memoir of advancing into old age as an unmarried, childless woman. Unsentimental, intelligent, unflinching and uplifting.

  bit.ly/1axUUCJ
  www.grantabooks.com/Diana-Athill

- Williamson, M. (2008) *The Age of Miracles: Embracing the New Midlife.* UK: Hay House

  As the Boomers move into their 60s they have a wholly different attitude to ageing. Williamson has a daughter but is interested in the whole range of what it means to be a middle-aged and older woman not just from the perspective of being a mother.

  bit.ly/18aTnOW
  www.marianne.com

On doing your grief work

- Beattie, M. (1990) *The Language of Letting Go*. USA: Hazelden
  This is a little book of daily readings on 'letting go'. It was written for co-dependents, but I find it incredibly useful for dealing with loss, change and grief. I've been referring to it regularly for over ten years.
  bit.ly/137MrfA
  www.melodybeattie.net

- Beattie, M. (2006) *The Grief Club: The Secret for Getting Through All Kinds of Change*. Minnesota, USA: Hazelden
  Apart from the (to me) *astonishing* omission of childlessness except due to abortion, miscarriage, stillbirth, infertility or bereavement from a list of more than 500 'losses' in her 'Master Loss Checklist', this is an excellent book from a woman whose writing has taught me so much about grief work and self-compassion. The website that accompanies the book has a grief forum which is free to join.
  bit.ly/16x94wq
  www.melodybeattie.net

- Chodron, P. (1997) *When Things Fall Apart: Heart Advice for Difficult Times*. USA: Shambala Publications
  The best book to turn to when you don't know where to turn. The first 'spiritual' book I ever read and still the best. You don't need to be a Buddhist to find great comfort in Pema's wise, funny and compassionate writing. I also recommend audio book versions read by her – she has a wonderfully warm and self-deprecating style and yet conveys great compassion towards her own, and all, our frailties as human beings.
  bit.ly/15mmmMU
  www.pemachodronfoundation.org

- Kübler-Ross, E. and Kessler, D. (2005) *On Grief and Grieving: Finding the Meaning of Grief Through the Five Stages of Loss.* London: Simon & Schuster

  This book is an excellent, humane and moving guide to the experience of grief. Although it doesn't address childless-related grief directly, it helped me to understand Kübler-Ross' Five Stages of Grief model.

  bit.ly/134DyrB

  www.ekrfoundation.org

On understanding and embracing your Inner Bitch

- Brown, B. (2010) *The Gifts of Imperfection: Let Go of Who You Think You're Supposed to Be and Embrace Who You Are.* USA: Hazelden Publishing

  This book contains quite a lot of references to parenting (slightly too many in my opinion!) but it's worth seeing past that to explore how Brené Brown, with her decades of research into shame and vulnerability, explores how to become a more 'wholehearted' person and work with our imperfections.

  bit.ly/11ImXvt

  www.brenebrown.com

- Ford, D. (2001) *Dark Side of the Light Chasers: Reclaiming Your Power, Creativity, Brilliance and Dreams.* London, UK: Hodder

  A truly terrible title for a truly wonderful book! Debbie Ford brought the Jungian concept of the 'Shadow' into the modern day with her work. Reading this book was the beginning, for me, of building a functional relationship with my Inner Bitch, and embracing my darkness as well as my light.

  bit.ly/18dnHMe

  www.debbieford.com

- Neff, K. (2011) *Self Compassion: Stop Beating Yourself Up and Leave Insecurity Behind.* UK: Hodder and Stoughton

  This book is an excellent guide to why beating yourself up doesn't work, why we do it – and what to do differently. Informative, practical and easy to read and implement.

  bit.ly/11VYgvH

  www.self-compassion.org

On forgiving your body

- Brown, B. (2007) *I Thought It Was Just Me: Making the Journey from "What Will People Think" to "I Am Enough".* USA: Gotham Books

  Brené Brown's first book and a very thorough and helpful analysis of both what shame is, and how to develop 'shame resilience'.

  bit.ly/18kSlzL

  www.brenebrown.com

- Brown, B. (2012) *Listening to Shame* [Online Video]. Available at: http://www.ted.com/talks/brene_brown_listening_to_shame.html (Accessed: May 2013)

  Only 20 minutes long but Brené makes such a difficult topic funny and affirming.

- Roth, G. (2011) *Women, Food & God: An Unexpected Path to Almost Everything.* UK: Simon and Schuster

  If you're an emotional eater, Geneen Roth's work is very illuminating. I also like her earlier book, *When You Eat At The Refrigerator, Pull Up a Chair (2006)*

  bit.ly/18aWeY6

  www.geneenroth.com

- Wolf, N. (1998) *The Beauty Myth: How Images of Beauty are Used Against Women.* UK: Vintage Books

  One of the main reasons I stopped reading women's magazines over a decade ago.

  bit.ly/15mCjCH

  www.naomiwolf.org

- Zackheim, V. (2007) Ed. *For Keeps: Women Tell the Truth About Their Bodies, Growing Older, and Acceptance.* UK: Avalon Publishing Group

  The real deal – real women's stories about real women's bodies.

  bit.ly/18RK4pJ

  www.victoriazackheim.com

On meaning, purpose, happiness and choices

- Beck, M. (2001) *Finding Your Own North Star: How to Claim the Life You Were Meant to Live.* London: Piatkus Books

  This is an overlong and rather frenetic read but has excellent exercises. Martha's blog is really worth subscribing to as well – I find her work is actually more digestible in smaller chunks.

  bit.ly/15BFUPE

  www.marthabeck.com

- Frankl, V. (1946) *Man's Search for Meaning.* London, UK: Ebury Publishing

  I've read it so many times and gifted it even more. A truly inspirational and life-changing book that can be read in an afternoon.

  bit.ly/13TH8a2

  Link to free PDF download of book: bit.ly/jbzbHF

- Ricard, M. (2006) *Happiness: A Guide to Developing Life's Most Important Skill.* London, UK: Atlantic Books

  An excellent guide to both spiritual and scientific approaches to understanding why happiness eludes so many of us and what we can practically do about it.

  bit.ly/10QRsg9

  www.en.wikipedia.org/wiki/Matthieu_Ricard

- Salecl, R. (2010) *Choice.* London: Profile Books.

  A short and very readable book on why choice, which is considered to be such a 'good' thing can also make us anxious wrecks!

  bit.ly/11IsYse

  An animated version of a talk she gave on 'Choice' at the RSA in London: bit.ly/130f4Nl

- Ditzler, J. (1994) *Your Best Year Yet: The 10 Questions that will change your life forever.* London, UK: Harper Element

  A short but rambling book about a rather brilliant system for working out what's working in your life and what's not, and how to set goals for the next 12 months to get yourself back on track.

  bit.ly/13WssFw

- Dickson, M. (2010) *Please Take One: One Step Towards a More Generous Life.* London: The Generous Press

  The book that launched a 'generosity movement' from the Founder of The Rainmaker Foundation in London. Simple ways to make the world a better place and yourself a whole lot happier.

  www.pleasetakeonestep.com

On developing your creativity (and dealing with the gremlins!)

- Cameron, J. (1995) *The Artist's Way: A Course in Discovering and Recovering Your Creative Self*. London, UK: Pan Books.

  Perhaps the very best book for getting going again if you want to rediscover the creative part of yourself. And we all have a creative part! Fantastic exercises, really well written and organised, tested over time and loved by millions of readers. Also a great online course available to work through the chapters.

  bit.ly/12ISSH7
  www.juliacameronlive.com

- Lamott, A. (2008) *Bird by Bird: Some Instructions on Writing and Life*. USA: Scribe Publications

  My favourite 'how to write' book and the one that got me writing again after my divorce. Wise, irreverent and brief – so you can't use it as an excuse not to get on and write…

  bit.ly/18b0ExY
  www.facebook.com/AnneLamott

- McNiff, S. (1998) *Trust the Process: An Artist's Guide to Letting Go*. USA: Shambala Publications

  A practical book with an esoteric flavour to help you get your creative juices flowing again. Examples from the visual arts, dramatic arts and writing but don't let that put you off. If the week-by-week approach of *The Artist's Way* is a bit too structured for you, try this.

  bit.ly/11IxsPo

- Pressfield, S. (2003) *The War of Art: Break Through the Blocks and Win Your Inner Creative Battles.* UK: Orion

  If you like your creative advice to be a bit 'muscular' and 'just do it' then Steven Pressfield will do it for you. His concept of 'resistance' has been very helpful for me in understanding why sometimes I'll do *anything* rather than get on with my writing or other creative projects. Lots of resources on his website too if you're looking for procrastination material.

  bit.ly/13FfNtk

  www.blackirishbooks.com

On thinking about changing your work/career as part of your Plan B

- Krznaric, R. (2012) *How to Find Fulfilling Work: The School of Life.* London, UK: Macmillan

  In the crowded field of 'career advice' this book stands out as a thoughtful yet immensely practical addition. I've read a *lot* of books in this area, but would recommend very few. This is one of them.

  bit.ly/178AZ8a

  www.romankrznaric.com

- Williams, J. (2010) *Screw Work Let's Play: How to Do What You Love and Get Paid for It.* London, UK: Pearson Business

  John Williams' book is the *first* one I recommend to Plan Bs who say they 'don't know what they want to do' *and* that 'they don't have time to do it' – usually in the same breath. His online '30 Day Challenge' is a really fun way to kick-start and test-drive a new idea without leaving your job or buying a camper van. Doing the challenge in 2011 gave me the impetus I needed to create the first version of the Gateway Women website.

  bit.ly/18dvNEG

  www.screwworkletsplay.com

- Williams, N. (1999) *The Work We Were Born to Do: Find the Work You Love, Love the Work You Do.* Kent, UK: Balloon View Publishing.

  Generous, wise and inspiring, Nick's books and the organisation he founded around it are the very best if you're looking to create a way to make a living that you love in the area of human potential. I've done some of his programmes and he helped me bring the Gateway Women concept to life and to nurture it (and me) through a time of great financial and emotional uncertainty for which I'll always be grateful.

  bit.ly/1buslnI

  www.inspired-entrepreneur.com

- Williams, N. (2011) *The Business You Were Born to Create*

  Free download at www.inspired-entrepreneur.com

Other women's stories

- Black, R. and Scull, L. (2005) *Beyond Childlessness: For Every Woman Who Wanted To Have a Child – and Didn't.* UK: Rodale Books.

  An early and important book from two British authors who between them interviewed countless others.

  bit.ly/12waGnK

  www.beyondchildlessness.com

- Carter, J. W. and Carter, M. (1998) *Sweet Grapes: How to Stop Being Infertile and Start Living Again.* USA: Perspectives

  This book was written by an infertile couple who took the decision together to 'stop being infertile' and instead to embrace a 'childfree life'. It's been recommended to me many times.

  bit.ly/11Wkn59

- De Ridder, N. and Nick W. (2013) *Just The Two of Us: Giving New Meaning to Our Lives Through Dealing with Infertility.* UK: Epubli

This book was written by a couple a few years after stopping infertility treatments. It's a guide for couples struggling to pick up their normal lives again. The book is both honest and uplifting and being so recent, resonates with a lot of readers.

bit.ly/11IhTC7
www.facebook.com/PastInfertility

- Fagalde Lick, S. (2012) *Childless by Marriage* US: Blue Hydrangea Productions

Writer and musician Sue Fagalde Lick's memoir and blog about life as a childless stepmother and now as a childless widow living on her own in her early 60s. An excellent insiders' view of a very difficult situation that so many childless-by-circumstance women are expected to take on the chin without minding!

http://bit.ly/12wkSxO
www.childlessbymarriage.blogspot.com.au

- Manterfield, L. (2010) *I'm Taking My Eggs and Going Home: How One Woman Dared to Say No to Motherhood.* USA: Steel Rose Press

This award-winning memoir of surviving and thriving after unsuccessful infertility treatment is bold, frank and gutsy. Lisa also went on to create the 'Life Without Baby' website and runs online workshops along with an online community.

bit.ly/12HlOOE
www.lifewithoutbaby.com

- Mahoney Tsingdinos, P. (2010) *Silent Sorority: A (Barren) Woman Gets Busy, Angry, Lost and Found.* USA: Booksurge Plc

  An award-winning infertility survivor's memoir – an 'alternative to the momoir' as Pamela puts it. A wry and intelligent read about infertility – and after.

  bit.ly/1blqtzi
  www.silentsorority.com

- Walker, E. L. (2011) *Complete Without Kids: An Insider's Guide to Childfree Living by Choice or by Chance.* Austin, USA: Greenleaf Book Group Press.

  The first book I read on life without children and a good introduction to the very different mindsets of childless vs. childfree people. Its strength is how many stories and interviews it contains.

  bit.ly/177aBAd
  www.completewithoutkids.com

- Yvette, P., Ann, R. and Lynne, J. (2012) *Being Fruitful Without Multiplying: Stories and Essays from Around the World.* Seattle, USA: Coffeetown Enterprises.

  This book is a mixture of childless *and* childfree women's stories from the US and other cultures around the world, although the emphasis is more towards childfree-by-choice women.

  bit.ly/15ADEID
  Coffeetown Press: bit.ly/1aseblN

ACKNOWLEDGMENTS

My thanks to each of you who financially supported the production of this book via crowdfunding and personal donations, including:

Alicia Cowan, Alison Heatherington, Amber Bielby, Anita Gaspar, Barbara Defrise Carter, Carol Cook, Cath Weeks, Christopher Hill, Claire Lloyd, Debs O'Donovan, Diane Osgood, Em Issatt, Emily Parikh, Fiona Hamilton, Gayathri Chidambi, Genny Swallow, Gill Lenton, Gina Whitsel, Helen Mills, Helen Acton, Helen Louise Jones, Irina Arcas, Jacqui Baverstock, Jen Thomas, Jennifer Barrett, Jennifer Richardson, Kabuki Snyder, Karen Schultz, Karen Ingala Smith, Kate Gilmore, Kathryn Penn, Katrina Berry, Kylie Bevon, Lara Vandalay, Laura Bernay, Leigh James, Liz Skinner, Lucy Firmin, Lynn Valentine, Marjon Bakker, Marlyn Hyde, Meriel Whale, Nicola Chapman, Pamela Vasile, Paula Knight, Pippa Sterne, Sarah Heseltine, Sarah Purdue, Sinéad Stack aka Agent Amsterdam, Sophia Henderson, Sue Shearman, Suzanne Wilson, Tamara Margitic, Valerie James, Wendy Stoner and others who helped but preferred to remain anonymous. Thank you to each of you.

My professional thanks to

Anita Belli at Casa Creative for creating such a supportive environment to write in.

Dennis Cain, a gifted therapist who helped me so much during the darkest days of my transformation. He knows how the caterpillar feels!

Helen Carroll, for writing such a sensitive article about me for The Guardian and enabling so many women to find out about Gateway Women. bit.ly/1h4Wudu

Joanna Penn of The Creative Penn for being such a generous guide to the world of self-publishing. www.thecreativepenn.com

John Williams & Selina Barker of the 'Screw Work Let's Play' 30 Day Challenge in 2011 for giving me a 30-day deadline to get the first Gateway Women website live. www.screwworkletsplay.com/challenge

Nick Williams & Niki Hignett of Inspired Entrepreneur, who supported and encouraged me through a very wobbly patch in my life and believed in the idea of Gateway Women when my confidence was below basement level. www.inspired-entrepreneur.com

Simon Fairclough, for capturing a real 'Jody smile' in his photograph of me.

The teaching staff and my fellow students at Terapia Institute, in particular Bozena Merrick and Lizzie Smosarski, and to Clare Soloway, for opening my heart and mind to the power of grief work. www.terapia.co.uk

And my personal thanks to

Elly & Mark, for their belief in me and for the priceless gift of somewhere to call home again.

Alexis Walters, for proofreading the manuscript and memories of the Lakes.

Anna Kendall, for being there from the caterpillar onwards.

Chloe Cunningham, for all the years since we shared that freezing changing room.

Christian, for reading the manuscript and staying alive.

Diana Weir, for a late and great proof-read with her legal eagle eye.

Diane Osgood, for LH and for *that* conversation in a coffee bar in South Kensington that helped me to see the bigger picture for GW.

Helen Burke and Jacqui Baverstock: 'the roomies', for their practical and emotional support. Carol Cook and Olivia Woodhouse for creating such a rocking Bristol Chapter of GW.

The deF's and the Newts. For being the best outlaw family a divorcee could wish for.

Janet Murray (SS), for her infectious enthusiasm and for repeatedly lending her cottage to ZZ and me for 'us' to write in. Thanks to James and Ben too for letting me steal their bedrooms.

Jo Foulkes, for reading an early manuscript and giving such helpful (and typewritten!) feedback.

Jo Wyeth, for so much love and support over so many years. And to both Jo and Will for having me to stay during those first few shaky post-divorce months.

Lumai, Harry and Eric, for being my god-children. And of course their parents Michele & Nathalie, Will & Jo, and Nunzio & Sophie for making that possible.

Mark Luscombe-Whyte and Marie Valenci, for food, sun, support and friendship.

Mike Dickson, for believing in me when I was struggling to agree

Peter Vrabel, for his grounded presence and for being such a good friend and protector to ZZ and me.

Sam Hunter, for being such a wise wolf. And the wee boss of course!

Stella Michael, for being Gateway Women's 'Godmother' and for believing, supporting and guiding both me and my ideas through the last few years.

The pioneering women of the very first Gateway Women Group: Stella, Genny, Fiona and Emma

Valerie James, for her twinkly intelligence, friendship and support.

ZZ, the magical cat, for coming home after eight years.

ENDNOTES

ALL THESE ENDNOTES ARE ALSO ACCESSIBLE ONLINE AS A LISTLY LIST AT BIT.LY/IAEMUMP

Chapter 1: Behind Every Woman Without Children is a Story

1   Office for National Statistics (UK) *Cohort Fertility* 2010 [Online] Available at:http://www.ons.gov.uk/ons/rel/fertility-analysis/cohort-fertility--england-and-wales/2010/cohort-fertility-2010.html (Accessed: May 2013)

2   Masters, J. (2006) *I never chose to be childless. I just never reached the let's-make-babies stage with anyone. Even when I was married'* The Observer, Sunday 12 March http://www.guardian.co.uk/lifeandstyle/2006/mar/12/features.woman7

3   Lehrer, J. (2007) *Proust Was a Neuroscientist.* New York: Houghton Mifflin Harcourt.

4   Rukeyser, M. (1968) *The Speed of Darkness.* In *Out of Silence: Selected Poems by Muriel Rukeyser.* USA: North-western University Press (Dec 1992)

Chapter 2: You're Not the Odd One Out

5   Office for National Statistics (UK) *ibid.*

6   Frejka, T. (2008) *Completed family size in Europe: Incipient decline of the two-child family model?* Demographic Research, Volume (19) pp.47-72 http://www.demographic-research.org/volumes/vol19/4/19-4.pdf

7   Nicolson, V. (2007) *Singled Out: How Two Million Women Survived Without Men after the First World War.* UK: Viking

8.   Wikipedia (2013) *Combined oral contraceptive pill* [Online] Available at: http://en.wikipedia.org/wiki/Combined_oral_contraceptive_pill (Accessed May 2013)

9   Science Daily (2012) *Late Motherhood: A Selfish Choice?* [Online] Available at:http://www.sciencedaily.com/releases/2012/09/120903143056.htm (Accessed May 2013)

10   Hanisch, C. (1969) *The Personal Is Political, Notes from the Second Year: Women's Liberation.* (1970) ed. Koedt, A. and Firestone, S. [Online] Available at: http://www.carolhanisch.org/CHwritings/PIP.html (Accessed May 2013)

11   Cannold, L. (2005) *What, No Baby? Why women are losing the freedom to mother and how they can get it back.* Freemantle, Australia: Curtin University Books

12   Orange, R. (2012) *All dads together: my new life among Sweden's latte pappas,* The Observer. Sunday 18 November http://www.guardian.co.uk/money/2012/nov/18/swedish-latte-pappa-shared-childcare?INTCMP=SRCH

13   Doughty, S. (2013) *Long days at nursery or with childminders 'raising a generation of school tearaways'* The Daily Mail. Monday 11 March. http://www.dailymail.co.uk/news/article-2291323/Long-days-nursery-childminders-raising-generation-school-tearaways.html

Chapter 3: Motherhood with a capital 'M'

14   Wikipedia (2013) *Plato* [Online]. Available at: http://en.wikipedia.org/wiki/Plato (Accessed: May 2013)

15   Cusk, R. (2003) *A Life's Work: On Becoming A Mother.* UK: Picador

16 Cusk, R. (2008) *I was only being honest.* The Guardian, Friday 21 March. http://www.guardian.co.uk/books/2008/mar/21/biography.women

17 Arnold, L. and Campbell C. (2013) *The High Price of Being Single in America.* The Atlantic. Monday 14 January, 2013 http://www.theatlantic.com/sexes/archive/2013/01/the-high-price-of-being-single-in-america/267043/ (Accessed May 2013)

18 Spock, B. (1946) *The Common Sense Book of Baby and Child Care.* New York: Duell, Sloan and Pearce http://en.wikipedia.org/wiki/The Common Sense Book of Baby and Child Care (Accessed May 2013)

19 Kargmen, J. (2007) *Momzillas* London, UK: Harper Perennial

20 Carroll, L. (2012) *The Baby Matrix* USA: LiveTrue Books www.livetruebooks.com

21 Salecl, R. (2010) *Choice* London: Profile Books.

Chapter 4: Working through the Grief of Childlessness

22 Day, J. (2011) *Light at the End of the Tunnel,* Gateway Women, 5 April [Online]. Available at: http://gateway-women.com/2011/04/05/light-at-the-end-of-the-tunnel/ (Accessed: May 2013).

23 Wikipedia (2013) *Pregnancy over age 50* [Online] Available at: http://en.wikipedia.org/wiki/Pregnancy over age 50 (Accessed: May 2013)

24 Wikipedia (2013) *In Vitro Fertilization* [Online] Available at: http://en.wikipedia.org/wiki/In vitro fertilisation (Accessed: May 2013)

25 Kübler-Ross, E. (1969) *On Death and Dying.* New York: Routledge

26 Elisabeth Kübler-Ross Foundation (2013) *Welcome* [Online] Available at: http://www.ekrfoundation.org/ (Accessed: May 2013)

27 Sapsted, D., Foster, P. and Jones, G. (2011) *'Grief is price of love, says the Queen'* The Telegraph, Wednesday 21 September. http://www.telegraph.co.uk/news/worldnews/northamerica/usa/1341155/Grief-is-price-of-love-says-the-Queen.html

28 Beattie, M. (1990) *The Language of Letting Go.* USA: Hazelden

Chapter 5: Liberating Yourself From The Opinions of Others

29 Linder, D. (2012) Famous Trials, *Poems Written by Lord Alfred Douglas* [Online] University of Missouri-Kansas City (UMKC) School of Law. Available at: http://law2.umkc.edu/faculty/projects/ftrials/wilde/poemsofdouglas.htm (Accessed: May 2013)

30 Chocano, C. (2012) *Girls Love Math. We Never Stop Doing It.* The New York Times. November 16 [Online] Available at: http://www.nytimes.com/2012/11/18/magazine/girls-love-math-we-never-stop-doing-it.html?pagewanted=all&_r=2& (Accessed: May 2013)

31 Chocano, *ibid.*

32 Wroe, N. (2012) *Janet Baker: A life in music.* The Guardian, Friday 13 July. http://www.guardian.co.uk/culture/2012/jul/13/janet-baker-life-in-writing (Accessed: May 2013)

33 Carroll, H. (2012) I may not be a mother - but I'm still a person… *Irish Independent* [Online]. Available at: http://www.independent.ie/lifestyle/parenting/i-may-not-be-a-mother-but-im-still-a-person-3041601.html (Accessed: May 2013)

34 Savvy Auntie http://www.savvyauntie.com

35 Hilliard, C. (2012) *I'm Not A Lesbian, I'm Just Childless.* Huffington Post, 20 July [Online] Available at: http://www.huffingtonpost.com/Chlo%C3%A9%20Hilliard/not-lesbian-just-childless_b_1687646.html (Accessed: May 2013)

36 Fagalde Lick, S. (2012) *Childless by Marriage.* USA: Blue Hydrangea Productions http://www.childlessbymarriage.com

37 Green, J. (2000) *How Many Witches* [Online] Available at: http://www.holocaust-history.org/~rjg/witches.shtml (Accessed: May 2013)

38 Stavrakopoulou, F. (Forthcoming 2015) *Baal and Asherah: Image, Sex, Power, and the Other.* Oxford, UK: Oxford University Press. More: http://humanities.exeter.ac.uk/theology/staff/stavrakopoulou

39 Howard, S. (2012) *Kids: Who Needs Them? We NoMos – Not Mothers – Are Out and We are Proud and We're Busy Making Our Own Friends and Support Networks.* The Sunday Times Style Magazine. Sunday 6 May Available at: http://mantramanga.files.wordpress.com/2011/04/kids-who-needs-them.jpg

40 Day, J. (2012) *The Gateway Women Manifesto: Are Childless Women the New Suffragettes?* Gateway Women, 3 May [Online] Available at: http://gateway-women.com/2012/05/03/the-nomos-manifesto-are-childless-women-the-new-suffragettes/ (Accessed: May 2013)

Chapter 6: *Who Moved My Mojo?*

41 Robbins, T. (2006) *Why We Do What We Do* [online video] Available at: http://ow.ly/bEsgT (Accessed: May 2013)

42 Frankl, V. (1946) *Man's Search for Meaning.* Translated from German by I. Lasch. With a Preface by Gordon W. Allport and Preface to the 1992 Edition by V. Frankl (2004) London, UK: Ebury Publishing

Chapter 7: *Letting Go of Your Burnt Out Dreams*

43 Wikipedia (2013) *Combined oral contraceptive pill* [Online] Available at:http://en.wikipedia.org/wiki/Combined_oral_contraceptive_pill (Accessed May 2013)

44 Dr Phil (2013) *National Parenting Survey* [Online] Available at: http://www.drphil.com/articles/article/311 (Accessed May 2013)

45 Carroll, L. (2013) *Getting Real About Regret* [Online] Available at: http://lauracarroll.com/getting-real-about-regret/#sthash.5NsXwdS8.dpuf (Accessed May 2013)

Chapter 8: *Reconnecting to Your Source*

46 Brown, B. (2013) The Power of Vulnerability. Live talk at The RSA in London, UK http://www.thersa.org/events/audio-and-past-events/2013/the-power-of-vulnerability (Accessed July 2013)

47 de Chardin, P. T. (1955) *The Phenomenon of Man.* London, UK (1959): William Collins http://en.wikipedia.org/wiki/The_Phenomenon_of_Man

48 Cameron, J. (1995) *The Artist's Way: A Course in Discovering and Recovering Your Creative Self.* London, UK: Pan Books

49 Neff, K. (2011) *Self Compassion: stop beating yourself up and leave insecurity behind.* UK: Hodder and Stoughton

50. Brown, B. (2010) *The Gifts of Imperfection: Let Go of Who You Think You're Supposed to Be and Embrace Who You Are.* USA: Hazelden Publishing

51 Dickson, M. (2010) *Please Take One: Step Towards a More Generous Life.* London: The Generous Press

Chapter 9: The Mother Within

52 Neff, K. *ibid* pp47-49

53 Gottman, J. (1994) *Why Marriages Succeed Or Fail And How to Make Yours Last.* New York, USA: Simon & Schuster

54 Fredrickson, B. (2009) *Positivity: Groundbreaking Research Reveals How to Embrace the Hidden Strength of Positive Emotions, Overcome Negativity, and Thrive.* USA: Crown Publishing Group

55 Neff, K. *ibid*, pp50-51

56 Wikipedia (2013) *Donald Winnicott* [Online]. Available at: http://en.wikipedia.org/wiki/Donald_Winnicott (Accessed: May 2013)

57 Cameron, J *ibid.* www.juliacameronlive.com/basic-tools/morning-pages

Chapter 10: Creating a Life For Yourself as a Childless Woman

58 Cameron, J. *ibid.*

59 Wikipedia (2013) *Cyril Connolly* [Online]. Available at: http://en.wikipedia.org/wiki/Cyril_Connolly (Accessed: May 2013)

60 Woolf, V. (1942) *Professions for Women. Collected in Women in Writing* (2003) Ed. Michele Barrett. UK: Houghton Mifflin Harcourt

61 Cooke, R. (2012) *Jenny Saville: 'I want to be a painter of modern life, and modern bodies'* The Guardian. Saturday 9 June http://www.guardian.co.uk/artanddesign/2012/jun/09/jenny-saville-painter-modern-bodies (Accessed: May 2013)

62 Brown, S. (2008) *Play is more than fun* [Online Video] Available at: http://www.ted.com/talks/stuart_brown_says_play_is_more_than_fun_it_s_vital.html (Accessed: May 2013)

Chapter 11: Putting Your Plan B Together

63 Ehrenreich, B. (2010) *Smile or Die: How Positive Thinking Fooled America and the World.* UK: Granta Books

64 Wikipedia (2013) *Joseph Campbell* [Online] Available at: http://en.wikipedia.org/wiki/Joseph_Campbell#cite_note-50 (Accessed: May 2013)

65 Moyers, J. C. (1989) *Joseph Campbell: Follow Your Bliss Conversations With Bill Moyers.* USA: Harper Collins

66 Robbins, T. (2006) *Why We Do What We Do* [Online Video] Available at: http://ow.ly/bEsgT (Accessed: May 2013)

67 Robbins, T. *ibid.*

68 Wikipedia (2013) Maslow's hierarchy of needs [Online] Available at: http://en.wikipedia.org/wiki/Maslow%27s_hierarchy_of_needs (Accessed: May 2013)

69 Wikipedia (2013) *George E. P. Box* [Online] Available at: http://en.wikipedia.org/wiki/George_E._P._Box (Accessed: May 2013)

70 Pressfield, S. (2003) *The War of Art: Winning the Inner Creative Battle.* USA: Orion

Chapter 12: Taking Off the Invisibility Cloak

71 Steinem, G. (1971) *Sisterhood* New York Magazine, 20 December, p. 49 http://en.wikiquote.org/wiki/Gloria_Steinem

72 Brunel University London (2013) *Mary Pat Sullivan: Programme Leader* MA Social Work [Online] http://www.brunel.ac.uk/shssc/people/social-work/mary-pat-sullivan (Accessed: May 2013)

73 Pinterest (2013) *Gateway Women Childless and Childfree Role Models.* [Online] Available at: http://www.pinterest.com/gatewaywomen/gateway-women-childless-childfree-women-role-model/ (Accessed: October 2013)

74. Eshure – European Society of Human Reproduction and Embryology (2013) *Art Fact Sheet* [Online] Available at: http://www.eshre.eu/sitecore/content/Home/Guidelines%20and%20Legal/ART%20fact%20sheet (Accessed: Nov 2013)

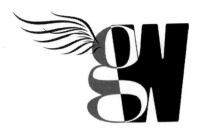

Thank you to all the women, all over the world, who have come into my life as a result of Gateway Women.

We may not be mothers but we're here,
we care, we count and we ROCK!!

For further information about Gateway Women workshops or events, to set up a GW reading group for this book in your area, or to join our free private online community, visit:

www.gateway-women.com